CONTENTS

SOUND SEARCH

SOUND SEARCH

A SPEECH AND LANGUAGE DRILLBOOK

Jerry Griffith and **Lynn E. Miner**

UNIVERSITY OF ILLINOIS PRESS
URBANA AND CHICAGO

Illini Books edition, 1986

This book is printed on acid-free paper.

Library of Congress Cataloging-in-Publication Data

Griffith, Jerry.
Sound search.

Rev. ed. of: Phonetic context drillbook. c1979.
Materials in this book are also available in software format for use with the personal computer.
Includes index.
1. Speech therapy—Exercises. I. Miner, Lynn E.
II. Griffith, Jerry. Phonetic context drillbook.
III. Title. [DNLM: 1. Phonetics. 2. Speech Therapy.
WM 475 G853s]
RC423.G74 1986 616.85′5′06 85-23224
ISBN 0-252-01326-3 (alk. paper) [Previously published by Prentice-Hall Inc. under ISBN 0-13-665361-7]

PREFACE

This drillbook provides an extensive source of words, phrases, and sentences for use by speech-language pathologists, students, and other professionals. The materials are based on a unique classification of the thousand most frequently used words, cross-referenced according to the major linguistic features typically used in clinical work, teaching, and research. The word lists are organized by

—phonemes: consonants, vowels, and diphthongs;
—syllable position: initial, medial, and final;
—syllable stress: stressed and unstressed;
—phonetic context: arranged for frequency of occurrence within phonemes;
—distinctive features: place and manner of production and voicing.

In addition to these multiple word lists, the drillbook also contains more than 6000 common phrases and sentences representing the phonetic contexts for all phonemes.

This book is primarily intended for the professional speech-language pathologist. Students preparing to be speech-language pathologists will find the materials particularly helpful in their clinical practicum experience. Other professionals who are concerned with speech, language, and language-related skills will also find the materials useful. This would include teachers of the acoustically handicapped, special education, learning disabilities, remedial reading, voice and diction, and phonetics. Researchers in speech-language pathology, audiology, psychology, psycholinguistics, education, and linguistics who wish to control the phonetic, syllabic, and word elements of language may refer to the word lists and frequency distributions.

For ease of reference and use, all phonemes are presented in the format described below:

/f/ PHONEME IDENTIFICATION

Distinctive Features: place and manner of production voicing.
/f/ International Phonetic Alphabet symbol for the phoneme, its phonetic context and a description of syllable position and syllable stress. Example:

/f/ ***vowel combinations:*** Initial position of a stressed syllable

Deep Test

/fi/ feel /fɪ/ fill /fe/ face /faʊ/ found

Since McDonald (1964) introduced the idea, it has become common practice to test articulation of a sound in a variety of words or "phonetic contexts." In this section there is an example of a word for each context that actually occurs for each phoneme. Four examples are shown above. These words will serve as a brief "deep test" to determine which context(s) may produce a correct production or the closest approximation of the sound. The contexts for each phoneme are identified using conventional phonetic transcriptions to represent "standard" pronunciations. Because phonetic transcription is not an exact science, there may be some dialect variations of a transcribed context.

Common Words

/fɪ/	/fe/	/fi/	/faʊ/
fifty	face	feel	found
figure	fail	feet	
fill	famous	field	
finger	favor		
finish			
fit			
fish			

In this section the contexts are shown in separate columns. Each column contains all of the common words which represent that context. It is obvious that there are more words for some contexts than for others. Consequently, it is possible to select from the more frequently spoken contexts.

Everyday Language

Phrases	Sentences
/fɪ/	
1. never fear	1. Never fear, ____ is here!
/fe/	
1. face him	1. How'll I face him?
fi/	
1. feel funny	1. I feel funny today.
/faʊ/	
1. found it	1. I found it!

This section contains five phrases and five related sentences for each phonetic context. One example for each of four contexts is shown above. They represent daily language common to both children and adults. Contemporary usage, idioms, and an occasional proverb are included. Slang and profanity have been avoided. For variety and motivation, some familiar phrases and quotations have been left incomplete to be filled in by the speaker. Some may stimulate additional conversation. None of the sentences is intentionally "loaded" with a sound. Real language is not constructed this way. The phrases may, of course, be used separately from the sentences. In fact, many additional sentences may be constructed from a phrase to suit individual needs.

Blends have been identified for each of the following consonants and a deep test, word lists, and phrases and sentences have been provided for each: /p, b, t, k, g, f, s, l, r, m, n, ŋ/. Blends are located at the end of the appropriate consonant section. For example, the /p/ blends are found following the /p/ vowel contexts. To avoid duplication, consonant blends are not listed under all members of the blend. For example, the /pl/ blends are listed only under /p/ and not under /l/. All blends, however, are cross-referenced by page number in the Index.

In the introductory chapter we will describe how the materials may be used in articulation therapy. Later we suggest some applications to other types of speech and language disorders. Nothing, however, can replace the ingenuity and adaptability of the creative professional who will use the best of materials only as a means to an end.

The materials in this book are also available in software format for use with personal computers. Table III (page 308) shows how the sounds have been grouped on seven disks. A disk contains all of the drillbook materials for a respective sound group, including the deep test, word lists, phrases, and sentences. To increase the effectiveness of the lists, each may be printed in a random sequence to prevent memory effects from repeated practice. In addition, the program allows the user to change or add words.

J.G.
L.E.M.

INTRODUCTION

All language units–phonemes, syllables, words, phrases, sentences–rank themselves for frequency of use or occurrence. This means that our language system is stable and orderly. Word frequency has been shown to be significantly related to a variety of speech and language disorders. Some of these relationships will be pointed out later in this chapter.

The contexts in the Drillbook are presented according to their comparative and absolute frequency of occurrence ranks. In addition, Table I and Table II are presented to show the frequency of occurrence of vowels, consonants, and diphthongs. The phoneme frequency ranks in Table I are derived from the words in the Drillbook. These words were taken from the language samples used by Thorndike and Lorge (1944) in compiling their frequency counts. Though there are many different lists of the most frequently used words, Dorn (1974) found a better than 90 percent duplication of words among these lists. Griffith and Miner (1973) transcribed the words and categorized them according to 16 linguistic variables using computer analysis techniques. For comparison purposes, the Tobias (1959) analysis, based on the word lists compiled by French, Carter, and Koenig (1930), is included in Table I. The Dorn and Tobias distributions are comparable and emphasize the relative stability of the phonological system. Almost equal numbers and essentially the same phonemes account for 50 percent of those used most often.

Table II shows the distribution of types of phonological syllables that occur in a spontaneous speech sample from normal and speech defective children. It should be noted that the most frequently used syllables are made up of no more than three phonetic elements. The contexts in the Drillbook are also identified according to syllable stress. Syllable stress combines with the

TABLE I. Rank order frequency of occurrence of 42 phonemes

Dorn (1974)		*Tobias (1959)*	
t		ɪ	
ɪ	4 = 27.94%	t	3 = 25.59%
n		ə	
r			
s		n	
d		d	
l	9 = 51.25%	s	9 = 50.09%
k		l	
ɛ		ð	
		ɪ	
ə			
m		m	
p		k	
ɚ		ɛ	
o	19 = 75.92%	w	
aɪ		aɪ	19 = 75.16%
b		j	
æ		ɔ	
e		z	
f		ɑ	
		æ	
i			
ɑ		e	
ɔ		o	
ʌ		i	
w		ɚ	
v		v	
g		ʊ	
u		h	
z		f	
h		b	
ʃ		g	
j	42 = 100%	p	
ŋ		ʌ	42 = 100%
aʊ		ŋ	
ð		u	
tʃ		θ	
ɝ		aʊ	
dʒ		ʃ	
θ		tʃ	
ʊ		ɝ	
ɔɪ		dʒ	
hw		hw	
ʒ		ɔɪ	
		ʒ	

Lists are in order of highest to lowest frequency.

Cumulative percent of frequency of occurrence is indicated.

TABLE II. Order and frequency of occurrence of phonologic syllables in American English

Syllables	*Percent*	*Total*
CV	32.40	
CVC	30.22	
VC	16.34	
V	8.11	87.07
CVCC	5.55	
CCVC	2.84	
CCV	2.64	
VCC	0.72	
CCVCC	0.60	
CCCVC	0.24	
CCCVCC	0.19	
CVCCC	0.12	
CCVCCC	0.02	
CCCV	0.01	12.93
All syllables	100.00	

From Faircloth, S. R., and M. A. Faircloth, *Phonetic Science: A Program of Instruction* (Englewood Cliffs, N.J.: Prentice-Hall, Inc., 1973), p. 78. Reprinted with permission.

syllable position of a sound (releasing or arresting) to have a facilitating effect on articulation performance (Faircloth & Faircloth, 1973; Schneider, 1973). Further, syllable stress contributes to *prosody,* a significant factor in the rapid sequencing of sounds and syllables in phrase patterns (Darley, Aronson, & Brown, 1975).

Tables I and II will serve as a guide for those who wish to work with the sounds and their phonetic contexts that are most frequently used. For example, correction of an articulation error on a sound that occurs often may result in more noticeable improvement in speech than correction of an error on an infrequent sound. Overall intelligibility would also be affected in cases of multiple articulation errors.

SUGGESTED PROCEDURE FOR ARTICULATION THERAPY

The materials in the Drillbook can be adapted to any articulation therapy method. However, it may be helpful to present a typical sequence that can be followed along with some reminders of techniques that may be useful to the learner.

Step 1. Identify the problem sound(s) by using an appropriate articulation test.

Step 2. Turn to each context for the problem sound and go through the "deep test" words. Use an imitative test method which has the learner repeat each word after the examiner. Since most therapy is designed around imitation of a stimulus word, this information is useful in anticipating responses to therapy.

Step 3. Keep in mind that better responses may occur in unstressed syllables.

Step 4. When the best context(s) are chosen, select the appropriate words for practice. As you examine these contexts, look for common characteristics such as releasing versus arresting position, stressed versus unstressed syllables, and vowel versus consonant blend contexts. You may find that a sound is most often correct when it arrests an unstressed syllable preceded by a particular vowel or the high front vowels. Look for similar characteristic patterns when selecting contexts for other phonemes. It is important to remember that it takes literally hundreds of correct productions of a sound to establish it as a speech habit. Keep careful records or charts to show how many times the sound has been practiced correctly. This is the key to carry-over.

Step 5. Now select the phrases and sentences that have been provided for further, more complex practice of the sound in its contexts. Correct articulation of a sound in connected speech is the final goal of therapy.

Step 6. When a phoneme is analyzed in a variety of contexts, it is likely that more than one context will result in an acceptable performance. This will also be true for more than one phoneme. For example, /r/ may be correct in some /r/ vowel contexts and in some /r/ consonant contexts. The speaker may practice correct productions and attempt new ones in both contexts. The same applies for different phonemes, i.e., more than one may be practiced in the same session. A good technique is to pair a correct context with a similar but incorrect one. If the speaker can produce /r/ in the word *reach,* pair it with words containing /r/ combined with the most adjacent vowel in the vowel progression, for example *rich.* If /s/ is correct in an /st/ blend, pair it with an /sl/ blend since use of the tongue tip is a characteristic of the correct context.

APPLICATION TO OTHER DISORDERS

The preceding series of steps describes a procedure to be followed in correcting individual sounds. Articulation errors may be found in many disorders and handicaps. Cleft palate speech, for example, is subject to co-articulation effects. Careful and thorough analysis of cleft palate speech in a wide variety of phonetic contexts will yield valuable information concerning articulatory gestures, velo-pharyngeal competency, acoustic hypernasality, and nasal air escape. It is possible to determine those contexts that tend to minimize these characteristics of cleft palate speech. It is recommended that essentially the steps outlined above be followed when evaluating and treating this type of disorder.

The materials in this book are appropriate to other types of disorders and they may be effective in bringing about early success in therapy, increasing motivation, and facilitating other aspects of language behavior.

Aphasia, Apraxia, and Dysarthria

–The more frequently used words affect the aphasic's visual and auditory comprehension (Schuell, Jenkins, & Landis, 1961; Seigel, 1959);

–Many of these words are commonly used nouns and verbs that are needed to restore functional language;

–The phrases and sentences provide good models for patterning and recall in aphasia therapy;

–The words, phrases, and sentences readily serve as stimuli for restoring written language skills for the aphasic;

–Therapy for apraxia of speech must be phoneme centered and provide for practice of sounds in units of gradually increasing complexity (Darley, Aronson, & Brown, 1975);

–Therapy for dysarthria is best designed around contexts that allow for compensatory articulatory gestures when necessary; weak or paralyzed articulators can handle some contexts more easily than others; and these serve as effective starting places to restore articulation skills (Darley, Aronson, & Brown, 1975);

–Early success with the brain-damaged adult increases motivation and reduces the emotional impact of communication loss.

Voice Disorders

–Varying vowel contexts tend to affect perceived vocal quality (Rees, 1958);

–Consonant and vowel contexts may be selected that will increase anterior articulation and wider oral opening to improve resonance (Boone, 1977);

–Appropriate context selection will allow for emphasis on specific articulation features, i.e., increasing lip mobility by concentrating on the labial consonant contexts;
–The naturalness of the phrases and sentences provides meaningful material for practice in inflection, intonation, and stress patterns, as well as speaking rate and intensity;
–Using frequently occurring vocabulary may facilitate the construction of effective nucleus situations for carry-over training of new voice skills.

Alaryngeal Speech

–The most frequently used words and their associated phrases and sentences can easily be controlled for number of syllables;
–Methods of alaryngeal speech vary in effectiveness with different sounds and sound combinations (Moolenaar-Bijl, 1953; Diedrich & Youngstrom, 1966);
–Syllabic stress can be controlled;
–Listener confusion matrices can be constructed to analyze problems of intelligibility;
–Contexts can be selected which systematically influence air flow and air pressure requirements (Boone, 1977).

Stuttering

–Since stutterers tend to stutter more often on frequently occurring words, this feature of language should be controlled in constructing therapy materials (Brown, 1945; Wischner, 1956);
–It is possible to provide systematic practice on feared sounds and words by selecting them from the appropriate lists;
–Phrases and sentences provide a variety of materials for establishing baseline fluency rates and maintaining newly acquired fluency levels;
–Phrases and sentences provide opportunity for varying rate, inflection, intonation, and stress patterns;
–Careful selection of phonetic contexts may facilitate reduction of preforming of sounds and hard contacts and provide practice in easy initiation of speech segments.

Bilingual Speech and Instruction in English as a Second Language

–The use of frequently occurring vocabulary is fundamental to language acquisition;
–Phonetic contexts, phrases, and sentences provide a basis for developing materials for pronounciation practice;

–Phrases and sentences provide models for development of useful, every-day language expressions;
–Practice in appropriate inflection, intonation, stress, rate, and intensity patterns is available.

Aural Rehabilitation

–Phoneme centered therapy for speech conservation is possible through systematic control of phonetic contexts;
–Speechreading practice materials can be constructed to conform to the error patterns revealed by speechreading tests (Hutton, 1969);
–Phrases and sentences are appropriate for establishing correct inflection, intonation, stress, rate, and intensity patterns or to maintain them in speech conservation activities;
–Construction of practice materials for auditory training is possible by matching phonetic contexts with auditory discrimination test results.

Speech Improvement

–Classroom speech improvement activities at elementary, high school, and college levels can be constructed to emphasize specific sounds;
–Practice in pronunciation of frequently used words may aid in altering dialect patterns;
–Phrases and sentences provide materials for inflection, intonation, rate, stress, and intensity pattern practice;
–Correction of minor articulation differences may be facilitated through careful phonetic context analysis;
–Auditory training materials emphasizing specific sounds and sound contrasts can be readily constructed.

CARRYOVER OF NEW SPEECH SKILLS

Establishing new speech skills and developing their use in daily communication requires meaningful practice sessions. The motivation to continue systematic practice is increased when success comes early and something meaningful is learned. Some important points to remember to facilitate carryover are these:

–Drill means practice of *correct* response, not hit-or-miss repetition of word lists;
–To assure that a sufficient number of correct responses is being amassed, develop a system of counting correct responses that can be recorded for later reference;
–Provide a sufficient variety of stimuli to maintain interest;
–Use materials that gradually increase in complexity, providing a greater challenge to the learner.

There are many different approaches to the management of speech and language disorders and they are all effective at one time or another. Regardless of the procedures used, however, speech behavior is bound by the lawfulness of the language code. This Drillbook is an attempt to capitalize on this lawfulness and, hopefully, to make all procedures more efficient.

REFERENCES

BOONE, D. J. *The Voice and Voice Therapy* (Englewood Cliffs, N.J.: Prentice-Hall, Inc., 1977).

BROWN, S. F. "The Loci of Stutterings in the Speech Sequence." *Journal of Speech Disorders,* II (1945), 181-92.

DARLEY, F., A. ARONSON, and J. BROWN. *Motor Speech Disorders* (Philadelphia: W. B. Saunders Company, 1975).

DIEDRICH, W. M., and K. A. YOUNGSTROM. *Alaryngeal Speech* (Springfield, Ill.: Charles C. Thomas, Publisher, 1966).

DORN, J. "A Phonetic Context Analysis of General American Consonants and Vowels." Unpublished Master's Thesis (Charleston, Ill.: Eastern Illinois University, 1974).

FAIRCLOTH, S., and M. FAIRCLOTH. *Phonetic Science: A Program of Instruction* (Englewood Cliffs, N.J.: Prentice-Hall, Inc., 1973).

FRENCH, N., C. CARTER, Jr., and W. KOENIG, Jr. "The Words and Sounds of Telephone Conversations." *Bell System Technical Journal,* IX (1930), 290-324.

GRIFFITH, J., and L. MINER. *Reference Word Lists: Grade Levels One and Two* (Chicago: Bell and Howell Company, 1973).

GRIFFITH, J., and L. MINER. *Reference Word Lists: Grade Levels Three and Four* (Chicago: Bell and Howell Company, 1973).

GRIFFITH, J., and L. MINER. *Reference Word Lists: Grade Levels Five and Six* (Chicago: Bell and Howell Company, 1973).

GRIFFITH, J., and L. MINER, *Reference Word Lists: Grade Levels Seven and Eight* (Chicago: Bell and Howell Company, 1973).

GRIFFITH, J., and L. MINER, *Reference Word Lists: Grade Levels Nine Through Twelve* (Chicago: Bell and Howell Company, 1973).

HUTTON, C. L. "Aural Rehabilitation," Chapter 5 in Griffith, J., ed., *Persons with Hearing Loss* (Springfield, Ill.: Charles C. Thomas, Publisher, 1969).

MCDONALD, E. *Articulation Testing and Treatment: A Sensory Motor Approach* (Pittsburgh: Stanwix House, 1964).

MOOLENAAR-BIJL, A. "The Importance of Certain Consonants in Esophageal Voice after Laryngectomy." *Annals of Otology, Rhinology and Laryngology,* LXII (1953), 979-89.

REES, M. "Some Variables Affecting Perceived Harshness." *Journal of Speech and Hearing Research,* I (1958), 155-68.

SCHNEIDER, C. "Phonetic Context and Articulation Ability." Unpublished Master's Thesis (Charleston, Ill.: Eastern Illinois University, 1973).

THORNDIKE, E., and I. LORGE. *The Teacher's Word Book of 30,000 Words* (New York: Teacher's College, Columbia University, 1944).

TOBIAS, J. "Relative Occurrence of Phonemes in American English." *Journal of the Acoustical Society of America,* XXXI (1959), 631.

SCHUELL, H., J. JENKINS, and L. LANDIS. "Relationship Between Auditory Comprehension and Word Frequency in Aphasia." *Journal of Speech and Hearing Research,* IV (1961), 30-36.

SIEGEL, G. M. "Dysphasic Speech Responses to Visual Word Stimuli." *Journal of Speech and Hearing Research,* II (1959), 152-60.

WISCHNER, G. J. "An Experimental Study of Some Verbal Cues as Instigators to Stuttering Behavior." Unpublished manuscript, University of Pittsburgh, 1956, cited in Brutten, E., and D. Shoemaker, eds., *The Modification of Stuttering* (Englewood Cliffs, N.J.: Prentice-Hall, Inc., 1967).

PHONETIC CONTEXTS

CONSONANTS

/p/ CONTEXTS

Distinctive features: bilabial, plosive, voiceless
/p/ ***vowel combinations:*** Initial position of a stressed syllable

Deep Test

/pi/ peace	/pɛ/ pear	/po/ post	/pʌ/ public	/pɔɪ/ point
/pɪ/ pick	/pæ/ pass	/pɑ/ part	/pɝ/ person	/paʊ/ power
/pe/ paid	/pʊ/ pull			

Common Words

/pe/	/pɪ/	/pɑ/	/pæ/	/po/	/pi/
page	appear	department	pass	post	peace
paid	opinion	part	passage	report	people
pain	period	party	past	support	piece
paint	pick	upon	path	suppose	
paper	picture	possible			
pay					

/pɛ/	/pʊ/	/pɝ/	/paʊ/	/pʌ/	/pɔɪ/
pear	pull	person	pound	public	point
prepare	put	purpose	power		

Everyday Language

Phrases

/pe/

1. first page
2. been paid
3. for the pain
4. paper come
5. pay the check

Sentences

1. Start on the first page.
2. Have you been paid?
3. Take something for the pain.
4. Has the paper come?
5. I'll pay the check.

Phrases	*Sentences*
/pɪ/	
1. pick it	1. Pick it up.
2. going period	2. I'm not going, period!
3. your opinion	3. That's your opinion.
4. get the picture	4. Do you get the picture?
5. appear anytime	5. It could appear anytime.
/pɑ/	
1. great party	1. It's a great party.
2. upon her return	2. Upon her return we can leave.
3. what part	3. What part do you play?
4. one part	4. One part is missing.
5. right department	5. You're in the right department.
/pæ/	
1. pass the butter	1. Pass the butter, please.
2. next passage	2. Read the next passage.
3. possible now	3. Anything is possible now.
4. past record	4. What's his past record?
5. the path	5. Show me the path.
/po/	
1. post office	1. Where's the post office?
2. the report	2. The report is ready.
3. your support	3. I'll need your support.
4. suppose he doesn't	4. Suppose he doesn't come?
5. report him	5. We'll report him absent.
/pi/	
1. peace and quiet	1. Oh for some peace and quiet!
2. funny people	2. They're funny people.
3. piece of your mind	3. Give him a piece of your mind.
4. some people	4. Some people don't care.
5. peace here	5. There's peace here.
/pɛ/	
1. in a pear tree	1. A partridge in a pear tree . . .
2. prepare to	2. Prepare to land!
3. prepare lunch	3. Can you prepare lunch?
4. like a pear	4. It's shaped like a pear.
5. apple or a pear	5. Do you want an apple or a pear?

Phrases	*Sentences*
/pʊ/	
1. pull on	1. Pull on this end.
2. put it in	2. Put it in the box.
3. put up	3. Put up or shut up!
4. put it off	4. Don't put it off.
5. some pull	5. He has some pull here.
/pɝ/	
1. one person	1. One person can do it.
2. the purpose	2. What's the purpose?
3. the chairperson	3. Who's the chairperson?
4. my purpose	4. My purpose is simple.
5. good person	5. She's a good person.
/paʊ/	
1. about a pound	1. It's about a pound.
2. the power	2. Turn on the power.
3. power failure	3. We had a power failure.
4. pound foolish	4. Penny wise, pound foolish.
5. lost a pound	5. Oh, I lost a pound!
/pʌ/	
1. public property	1. This is public property.
2. to the public	2. It's open to the public.
3. public notice	3. Here's a public notice.
4. notary public	4. She's a notary public.
5. public library	5. The public library is open.
/pɔɪ/	
1. your point	1. What's your point?
2. point to it	2. Point to it for me.
3. small point	3. It's a small point.
4. point a little	4. Sharpen the point a little.
5. point the way	5. Point the way and I'll go.

/p/ CONTEXTS

Distinctive features: bilabial, plosive, voiceless
/p/ ***vowel combinations:*** Initial position of an unstressed syllable

Deep Test

/pe/ newspaper /pə/ purpose /pɚ/ paper

Common Words

/pə/	/pɚ/	/pe/
company	newspaper	newspaper
position	paper	
purpose	perhaps	

Everyday Language

Phrases	*Sentences*
/pə/	
1. having company	1. We're having company.
2. what position	2. What position do you play?
3. no purpose	3. There's no purpose.
4. two's company	4. Two's company, three's _____.
5. change position	5. Change position now.
/pɚ/	
1. in the newspaper	1. I saw it in the newspaper.
2. more paper	2. We'll need more paper.
3. perhaps we can	3. Perhaps we can, we'll see.
4. in the paper	4. Run an ad in the paper.
5. newspaper people	5. Newspaper people are crazy.
/pe/	
1. in newspaper	1. Wrap it in newspaper.
2. in the newspaper	2. Put it in the newspaper.
3. in the newspaper	3. I read it in the newspaper.
4. the newspaper	4. Call the newspaper about it.
5. has the newspaper	5. Has the newspaper come yet?

/p/ CONTEXTS

Distinctive features: bilabial, plosive, voiceless
/p/ *vowel combinations:* Final position of a stressed syllable

Deep Test

/ip/ deep /ep/ shape /ɑp/ top /op/ hope /up/ group /ʌp/ up
/ɪp/ lip /ɛp/ step

Common Words

/ap/	/ip/	/ɪp/	/ʌp/	/ep/	/æp/	/ɛp/	/op/
drop	deep	lip	cup	escape	captain	step	hope
proper	keep	ship	up	shape			
shop	sleep	trip					
stop							
top							

/up/
group

Everyday Language

Phrases	*Sentences*
/ap/	
1. drop it	1. Drop it, you're covered!
2. that shop	2. Is that shop open?
3. stop, look	3. Stop, look, and listen!
4. on top	4. You're on top now.
5. proper way	5. This is the proper way.
/ip/	
1. deep subject	1. That's a deep subject.
2. keep going	2. You have to keep going.
3. need sleep	3. I need sleep.
4. sleep now	4. Go to sleep now.
5. deep trouble	5. You're in deep trouble.
/ɪp/	
1. your lip	1. Button your lip!
2. ship out	2. Shape up or ship out!
3. take a trip	3. Let's take a trip.
4. ship it	4. Ship it to me C.O.D.
5. my lip	5. My lip hurts.
/ʌp/	
1. one cup	1. Put in one cup.
2. up to you	2. It's up to you.
3. cup and saucer	3. Put out a cup and saucer.
4. up to now	4. Up to now it's been OK.
5. cup your hands	5. Cup your hands around it.

Phrases	*Sentences*
/ep/	
1. can't escape	1. You can't escape.
2. shape up	2. Shape up or _____.
3. good shape	3. It's in good shape.
4. what a shape	4. Wow, what a shape!
5. narrow escape	5. It was a narrow escape.
/æp/	
1. who's captain	1. Who's captain of the team?
2. team captain	2. You're the team captain.
3. ship's captain	3. Call the ship's captain.
4. the captain	4. Ask the captain first.
5. one captain	5. We can have only one captain.
/ɛp/	
1. first step	1. What's the first step?
2. step right	2. Step right up!
3. step down	3. Step down carefully.
4. your step	4. Watch your step.
5. step lively	5. Step lively now!
/op/	
1. give up hope	1. Don't give up hope.
2. I hope	2. I hope you can.
3. hope springs	3. Hope springs eternal!
4. hope so	4. We hope so.
5. little hope	5. They have little hope.
/up/	
1. the group	1. Join the group!
2. which group	2. Which group do you mean?
3. men's group	3. I mean the men's group.
4. women's group	4. Is there a women's group?
5. any group	5. Any group will do.

/p/ CONTEXTS

Distinctive features: bilabial, plosive, voiceless
/p/ ***blends:*** Initial position of a stressed syllable

Deep Test

/pl/ plan

Common Words

/pl/

complete
plan
plant

Everyday Language

Phrases	*Sentences*
/pl/	
1. all complete	1. Now it's all complete.
2. plan for tonight	2. What's the plan for tonight?
3. plant it here	3. Just plant it here.
4. a complete set	4. This is a complete set.
5. your plant	5. Your plant needs water.

/p/ CONTEXTS

Distinctive features: bilabial, plosive, voiceless
/p/ ***blends:*** Final position of a stressed syllable

Deep Test

/pt/ kept /ps/ perhaps

Common Words

/pt/	/ps/
accept	perhaps
except	
kept	

Everyday Language

Phrases	*Sentences*
/pt/	
1. I accept	1. I accept the challenge.
2. except me	2. There's no one here except me.
3. we kept	3. We kept regular hours.
4. kept it	4. I think he kept it.
5. accept it	5. Who'll accept it?

Phrases	*Sentences*
/ps/	
1. perhaps we	1. Perhaps we can.
2. they will perhaps	2. They will, perhaps, when they know.
3. perhaps someone	3. Perhaps someone tattled!
4. be it perhaps	4. You'd like to be it, perhaps?
5. perhaps they will	5. Perhaps they will today.

/b/ CONTEXTS

Distinctive features: bilabial, plosive, voiced
/b/ ***vowel combinations:*** Initial position of a stressed syllable

Deep Test

/bi/ be	/bɛ/ bed	/bɔ/ born	/bʊ/ book	/bɝ/ bird	/baʊ/ about
/bɪ/ bit	/bæ/ back	/bo/ boat	/bʌ/ but	/baɪ/ by	/bɔɪ/ boy
/be/ bay	/bɑ/ body				

Common Words

/bɪ/	/bɛ/	/bæ/	/bo/	/bi/	/be/	/bʌ/
big	bear	back	board	be	baby	above
bill	bed	bag	boat	beat	base	but
bit	been	bank	both	being	bay	butter
build	best	battle				
building	better					
built						
business						
busy						

/bɑ/	/bɝ/	/baɪ/	/bɔ/	/bʊ/	/baʊ/	/bɔɪ/
body	bird	buy	born	book	about	boy
box	burn	by				

Everyday Language

Phrases	*Sentences*
/bɪ/	
1. busy day	1. It's a busy day.
2. big boy	2. He's a big boy now.
3. a bit scared	3. I'm not a bit scared.
4. they're building	4. They're building a new house.
5. quit the business	5. He quit the business today.
/bɛ/	
1. better watch	1. You'd better watch it.
2. that's the best	2. That's the best I can do.
3. where've you	3. Where've you been tonight?
4. get to bed	4. Let's get to bed.
5. as a bear	5. He's mean as a bear.
/bæ/	
1. right back	1. I'll be right back.
2. in the bag	2. It's in the bag now.
3. won the battle	3. Won the battle, but lost the war.
4. in the bank	4. It's like money in the bank.
5. new bag	5. Is that a new bag?
/bo/	
1. the board	1. The board is rotten.
2. big boat	2. That's a big boat.
3. both games	3. We lost both games.
4. both of us	4. You can count on both of us.
5. new board	5. A new board will fix it.
/bi/	
1. be funny	1. Don't be funny!
2. beat it	2. He told me to beat it.
3. she's being	3. She's being extra careful.
4. I'll be	4. I'll be darned!
5. you be	5. Where will you be?
/be/	
1. cry baby	1. Don't be a cry baby.
2. broad base	2. It has a broad base.
3. Moonlight Bay	3. Let's sing "Moonlight Bay."
4. cute baby	4. What a cute baby!
5. on the bay	5. She lives on the bay.

Phrases	*Sentences*
/bʌ/	
1. above it	1. Keep your head above it.
2. but don't	2. Do it but don't tell me.
3. the butter	3. Pass the butter, please.
4. peanut butter	4. I love peanut butter.
5. above all	5. Above all, be nice.
/bɑ/	
1. your hair body	1. It gives your hair body.
2. this box	2. This box is empty.
3. full box	3. We'll find a full box.
4. body beautiful	4. She's the body beautiful.
5. my body	5. My body is a wreck!
/bɝ/	
1. burn slowly	1. It'll burn slowly.
2. the bird house	2. Did you see the bird house?
3. slight burn	3. It's only a slight burn.
4. bird watcher	4. She's a bird watcher.
5. burn your bridges	5. Don't burn your bridges.
/baɪ/	
1. get by	1. I'll get by somehow.
2. buy it	2. Did you buy it?
3. by me	3. Come sit by me.
4. by the way	4. By the way, she's here.
5. buy your lunch	5. I'll buy your lunch today.
/bɔ/	
1. born yesterday	1. I wasn't born yesterday.
2. born rich	2. He was born rich.
3. were you born	3. Where were you born?
4. born free	4. "Born Free" is a song.
5. born today	5. The baby was born today.
/bʊ/	
1. good book	1. That's a good book.
2. which book	2. Which book is that?
3. last book	3. The last book he wrote.
4. first book	4. What was his first book?
5. his last book	5. The same as his last book.

Phrases	*Sentences*
/baʊ/	
1. about time	1. It's about time.
2. about finished	2. I'm about finished.
3. about two	3. We started about two.
4. the story about	4. What's the story about?
5. all about	5. It's all about love.
/bɔɪ)	
1. strange boy	1. He's a strange boy.
2. good boy	2. But he's a good boy.
3. boy or girl	3. Was it a boy or girl?
4. boy was	4. Boy, was she mad!
5. boy friend	5. Who's your boy friend?

/b/ CONTEXTS

Distinctive features: bilabial, plosive, voiced
/b/ ***vowel combinations:*** Initial position of an unstressed syllable

Deep Test

/bɪ/ begin /bɚ/ member /bə/ probably

Common Words

/bɪ/	/bɚ/	/bə/
baby	labor	husband
became	member	probably
become	neighbor	
before	remember	
began		
begin		
behind		
believe		
belong		
beside		
between		
beyond		

Everyday Language

Phrases	*Sentences*
/bɪ/	
1. before you go	1. Before you go, tell me.
2. believe it	2. I don't believe it.
3. between them	3. Put it between them.
4. this belong	4. Where does this belong?
5. can't begin	5. I can't begin to tell you.
/bɚ/	
1. remember you	1. She'll remember you.
2. hard labor	2. That's hard labor.
3. good neighbor	3. Be a good neighbor.
4. new member	4. She's a new member.
5. labor of love	5. It's a labor of love.
/bə/	
1. new husband	1. She has a new husband.
2. probably right	2. You're probably right.
3. probably go	3. I'll probably go along.
4. whose husband	4. Whose husband is he?
5. we're probably	5. We're probably too late.

/b/ CONTEXTS

Distinctive features: bilabial, plosive, voiced
/b/ ***vowel combinations:*** Final position of a stressed syllable

Deep Test

/ɑb/ job /ʌb/ club

Common Words

/ʌb/	/ɑb/
club	job
public	
subject	

Everyday Language

Phrases	*Sentences*
/ʌb/	
1. the club	1. Join the club!
2. made public	2. It'll be made public soon.
3. big subject	3. This is a big subject.
4. deep subject	4. That's a deep subject.
5. public place	5. Is this a public place?
/ɑb/	
1. big job	1. It's a big job.
2. good job	2. A good job is hard to find.
3. new job	3. How's your new job?
4. tough job	4. You have a tough job.
5. one job	5. One job is enough.

/b/ CONTEXTS

Distinctive features: bilabial, plosive, voiced
/b/ ***blends:*** Initial position of a stressed syllable

Deep Test

/br/ break   /bl/ blue

Common Words

/br/	/bl/
branch	black
break	blood
bridge	blow
bright	blue
bring	
broken	
brother	
brought	
brown	

Everyday Language

Phrases	*Sentences*
/br/	
1. oh, brother	1. Oh, brother, not another one!
2. who brought	2. Who brought the potato chips?
3. break it	3. Don't break it, it's mine.
4. branch out	4. You should branch out if you can.
5. it's broken	5. Too bad, it's broken.
/bl/	
1. black day	1. This is a black day!
2. blood ran cold	2. My blood ran cold!
3. it's a blow	3. It's a blow to him.
4. be blue	4. Don't be blue.
5. blow harder	5. You'll have to blow harder.

/b/ CONTEXTS

Distinctive features: bilabial, plosive, voiced
/b/ ***blends:*** Initial position of an unstressed syllable

Deep Test

/bl/ probably

Common Words

/bl/

probably
problem

Everyday Language

Phrases	*Sentences*
/bl/	
1. probably win	1. They'll probably win.
2. probably so	2. It's probably so.
3. probably be here	3. He'll probably be here.
4. your problem	4. What's your problem?
5. big problem	5. You've got a big problem!

/t/ CONTEXTS

Distinctive features: linguaalveolar, plosive, voiceless
/t/ ***vowel combinations:*** Initial position of a stressed syllable

Deep Test

/ti/ teach	/tɛ/ tell	/tɔ/ tall	/tʊ/ took	/tɝ/ turn	/taɪ/ tie
/tɪ/ till	/tɑ/ top	/to/ told	/tu/ too	/tʌ/ touch	/taʊ/ town
/te/ take					

Common Words

/te/	/tɛ/	/tɪ/	/taɪ/	/tu/	/ti/	/tɔ/
contain	attempt	continue	tie	to	teach	talk
obtain	attention	material	time	too	teacher	tall
table	tear	till	tire	two		
take	tell	until	type			
taken						
taste						

/tɝ/	/tɑ/	/to/	/tʊ/	/tʌ/	/taʊ/
return	top	told	took	touch	town
turn					

Everyday Language

Phrases	*Sentences*
/te/	
1. set the table	1. Please set the table.
2. take turns	2. Let's take turns now.
3. I've taken	3. I've taken that course.
4. taste good	4. That doesn't taste good.
5. obtain a permit	5. You'll have to obtain a permit.
/tɛ/	
1. an attempt	1. At least make an attempt.
2. attention everyone	2. Attention, everyone, attention!
3. it'll tear	3. It'll tear if you pull it.
4. only ten	4. Only ten more to do!
5. don't tell	5. Please don't tell her.

Phrases	*Sentences*
/tɪ/	
1. till now	1. Till now it worked.
2. continue tomorrow	2. We'll continue tomorrow.
3. good material	3. That's good material.
4. until you finish	4. You can't go until you finish.
5. more material	5. We need more material.
/taɪ/	
1. a tie	1. Let's get him a tie.
2. tire easily	2. I seem to tire easily.
3. type a letter	3. Can you type a letter?
4. what type	4. What type is it?
5. just tie	5. Just tie a loose knot.
/tu/	
1. too much	1. It's too much for me.
2. too tired	2. I'm too tired to think.
3. two will be	3. Two will be plenty.
4. half past two	4. It's half past two now.
5. time to go	5. Time to go, I guess.
/ti/	
1. your teacher	1. Who's your teacher?
2. I'll teach	2. I'll teach you.
3. can teach	3. We can teach each other.
4. be a teacher	4. Do you want to be a teacher?
5. teach him	5. That'll teach him a lesson.
/tɔ/	
1. stand tall	1. Stand tall, man.
2. don't talk	2. Don't talk so much.
3. lot of talk	3. It's just a lot of talk.
4. tall story	4. Sounds like a tall story.
5. tall timber	5. Now that's tall timber.
/tɝ/	
1. return it	1. Can you return it?
2. turn left	2. Turn left, then right.
3. turn to go	3. One more turn to go.
4. you return	4. When will you return?
5. return mail	5. It came by return mail.

Phrases	*Sentences*
/ta/	
1. top shelf	1. It's on the top shelf.
2. top dog	2. He's top dog now.
3. top of the world	3. I'm on top of the world!
4. like a top	4. I slept like a top!
5. top notch	5. You did a top notch job.
/to/	
1. I told	1. I told you so.
2. told you	2. Who told you first?
3. told me	3. No one told me.
4. they told	4. They told me no.
5. we told	5. We told them twice.
/tʊ/	
1. you took	1. You took your time.
2. who took	2. Who took my chair?
3. it took	3. It took more time.
4. I took	4. I took that course.
5. we took	5. We took a wrong turn.
/tʌ/	
1. touch me	1. Don't touch me!
2. light touch	2. Use a light touch.
3. touch it	3. Touch it if you want.
4. touch her	4. It would touch her deeply.
5. touch of winter	5. There's a touch of winter now.
/taʊ/	
1. came to town	1. He came to town today.
2. across town	2. She lives across town.
3. cross town	3. Is that a cross town bus?
4. downtown	4. Let's go downtown.
5. a town house	5. They live in a town house.

/t/ CONTEXTS

Distinctive features: linguaalveolar, plosive, voiceless
/t/ ***vowel combinations:*** Initial position of an unstressed syllable

Deep Test

/tɪ/ party /tu/ into /tɚ/ after /tə/ today /taɪ/ sometimes

Common Words

/tɪ/	/tɚ/	/tə/	/tu/	/taɪ/
article	after	distance	into	sometimes
beautiful	afternoon	important		
beauty	better	today		
captain	butter	together		
certain	center	tomorrow		
certainly	character			
duty	daughter			
fifty	doctor			
meeting	enter			
mountain	interest			
native	letter			
notice	master			
party	matter			
practice	quarter			
pretty	sister			
society	water			
system	winter			
thirty				
twenty				

Everyday Language

Phrases	*Sentences*
/tɪ/	
1. certain to	1. It's certain to rain.
2. native here	2. Are you a native here?
3. duty now	3. Do your duty now!
4. the party	4. Come to the party.
5. practice makes	5. Practice makes perfect!
/tɚ/	
1. after me	1. You're next after me.
2. your doctor	2. Who's your doctor?
3. off center	3. It's a little off center.
4. water the plants	4. Don't forget to water the plants.
5. a quarter	5. You owe me a quarter.

Phrases	*Sentences*
/tə/	
1. it's important	1. It's important to me.
2. today is	2. Today is the beginning.
3. tomorrow will tell	3. Tomorrow will tell the tale.
4. go together	4. Let's go together
5. quite a distance	5. That's quite a distance.
/tu/	
1. turn into	1. Turn into the drive.
2. into my coat	2. I can't get into my coat.
3. into town	3. Let's drive into town.
4. into the water	4. He jumped into the water.
5. into my lap	5. It fell into my lap.
/taɪ/	
1. sometimes I	1. Sometimes I wonder about you.
2. sometimes it does	2. Sometimes it does, sometimes not.
3. go there sometimes	3. We go there sometimes.
4. sometimes he stops	4. Sometimes he stops by here.
5. puzzles me sometimes	5. It really puzzles me sometimes.

/t/ CONTEXTS

Distinctive features: linguaalveolar, plosive, voiceless
/t/ ***vowel combinations:*** Final position of a stressed syllable

Deep Test

/it/ eat	/ɛt/ get	/ɔt/ ought	/ut/ suit	/aɪt/ height
/ɪt/ it	/æt/ at	/ot/ coat	/ɝt/ hurt	/aʊt/ out
/et/ eight	/ɑt/ hot	/ʊt/ put	/ʌt/ cut	

Common Words

/aɪt/	/it/	/et/	/ɪt/	/ɑt/	/ɛt/	/æt/
bright	beat	date	admit	cotton	forget	at
fight	complete	eight	bit	got	get	attribute
height	eat	gate	city	hot	let	fat
knight	feet	great	fit	lot	met	hat
light	heat	late	it	not	set	sat
might	meat	rate	little	shot	yet	that
night	meet	state	permit	spot		
quite	seat	straight	sit			
right	street	wait	written			
sight	sweet	weight				
white						
write						

/aʊt/	/ot/	/ɔt/	/ʌt/	/ʊt/	/ut/	/ɝt/
about	boat	brought	but	foot	fruit	hurt
doubt	coat	caught	cut	put	suit	
out	note	ought				
outside	vote					
shout	wrote					
without						

Everyday Language

Phrases	*Sentences*
/aɪt/	
1. on the light	1. Turn on the light.
2. be right	2. You may be right.
3. good night	3. Good night for now.
4. might be	4. I might be able to go.
5. in sight	5. There's no rain in sight.
/it/	
1. we meet	1. Where should we meet?
2. your seat	2. Take your seat.
3. the heat	3. Turn up the heat, please.
4. shall we eat	4. Where shall we eat?
5. my feet	5. My feet are cold.

Phrases	*Sentences*
/eɪt/	
1. be late	1. Don't be late.
2. have to wait	2. You'll have to wait.
3. late show	3. Did you see the late show?
4. your date	4. Who's your date tonight?
5. eight o'clock	5. It starts at eight o'clock.
/ɪt/	
1. sit by me	1. Come and sit by me.
2. have to admit	2. I'll have to admit I'm wrong.
3. little bit	3. Won't you have a little bit?
4. doesn't fit	4. This one doesn't fit.
5. is it	5. Is it time to go?
/ɑt/	
1. soft as cotton	1. It's soft as cotton.
2. a lot	2. I like you a lot.
3. that's not	3. That's not a good idea.
4. hot today	4. It's sure hot today!
5. take a shot	5. I'll take a shot at it.
/ɛt/	
1. better get	1. He better get busy.
2. don't forget	2. Don't forget the party.
3. let me	3. Let me help you.
4. we've met	4. We've met before.
5. you set	5. Will you set the table?
/æt/	
1. fat chance	1. Fat chance of winning now!
2. my hat	2. Who took my hat?
3. that does	3. That does it for now.
4. sat there	4. He just sat there.
5. at me	5. Don't stare at me!
/aʊt/	
1. about time	1. It's about time.
2. doubt it	2. I doubt it very much.
3. they're out	3. They're out of that kind.
4. stay outside	4. Stay outside the lines.
5. don't shout	5. Don't shout at me!

Phrases	*Sentences*
/ot/	
1. beautiful boat	1. That's a beautiful boat.
2. my coat	2. Have you seen my coat?
3. a note	3. We left them a note.
4. vote today	4. Did you vote today?
5. I wrote	5. I wrote it down.
/ɔt/	
1. he brought	1. He brought a friend.
2. she caught	2. She caught the biggest ones.
3. he ought	3. He ought to wait.
4. I thought	4. I thought you'd like it.
5. someone ought	5. Someone ought to say so.
/ʌt/	
1. but I	1. I would but I can't.
2. cut me	2. Cut me a small piece.
3. short cut	3. Do you know a short cut?
4. but me	4. Is there anyone but me?
5. cut it	5. Oh, cut it out!
/ʊt/	
1. put it	1. Put it over here.
2. by a foot	2. It's short by a foot.
3. on one foot	3. Stand on one foot.
4. put it in	4. Let's put it in the hole.
5. foot the bill	5. Who'll foot the bill?
/ut/	
1. new suit	1. Is that a new suit?
2. fresh fruit	2. Fresh fruit is best.
3. suit yourself	3. Suit yourself, but I'll go.
4. fruit juice	4. I'd like some fruit juice.
5. suit them	5. I hope that will suit them.
/ɝt/	
1. hurt you	1. It won't hurt you.
2. that hurt	2. Did that hurt?
3. little hurt	3. A little hurt is OK.
4. was hurt	4. No one was hurt.
5. that hurt	5. That hurt just a little bit.

/t/ CONTEXTS

Distinctive features: linguaalveolar, plosive, voiceless
/t/ ***vowel combinations:*** Final position of an unstressed syllable

Deep Test

/ɪt/ visit   /ət/ whatever

Common Words

/ɪt/	/ət/
minute	whatever
spirit	
visit	

Everyday Language

Phrases	*Sentences*
/ɪt/	
1. a minute	1. Wait a minute!
2. the spirit	2. That's the spirit!
3. brief visit	3. Make it a brief visit.
4. take a minute	4. I'll just take a minute.
5. when the spirit	5. When the spirit moves him, he will.
/ət/	
1. whatever happens	1. Whatever happens, don't quit.
2. whatever happened	2. Whatever happened to Bill?
3. whatever you say	3. Well, whatever you say.
4. whatever shall	4. Whatever shall we do?
5. whatever will	5. Who knows whatever will happen!

/t/ CONTEXTS

Distinctive features: linguaalveolar, plosive, voiceless
/t/ **blends**: Initial position of a stressed syllable

Deep Test

/tw/ twenty

Everyday Language

Phrases	*Sentences*
/tw/	
1. between terms	1. We're between terms.
2. almost twelve	2. It's almost twelve.
3. twenty more	3. Here are twenty more.
4. between meals	4. Don't eat between meals.
5. twelve more days	5. Twelve more days to go!

/t/ CONTEXTS

Distinctive features: linguaalveolar, plosive, voiceless
/t/ ***blends:*** Final position of a stressed syllable

Deep Test

/ts/ its

Common Words

/ts/

it's
its
that's

Everyday Language

Phrases	*Sentences*
/ts/	
1. it's a new	1. It's a new start.
2. its mother	2. Where's its mother?
3. that's all	3. That's all for now.
4. that's right	4. That's right, leave me!
5. that's the one	5. I imagine that's the one.

/d/ CONTEXTS

Distinctive features: linguaalveolar, plosive, voiced
/d/ ***vowel combinations:*** Initial position of a stressed syllable

Deep Test

/di/ deep	/dɛ/ dead	/dɔ/ dog	/dɝ/during	/daɪ/ die
/dɪ/ did	/dæ/ dance	/do/ door	/dʌ/ does	/daʊ/ doubt
/de/ day	/dɑ/ dollar	/du/ do		

Common Words

/dɪ/	/de/	/di/	/du/	/dʌ/	/dɛ/	/dɑ/
condition	daily	deal	do	does	dare	dark
dear	danger	deep	due	doesn't	dead	doctor
did	date	idea	duty	done	death	dollar
difference	day	indeed	produce	double		
different	today					
dinner						
distance						

/dɔ/	/do/	/daʊ/	/dæ/	/dɝ/	/daɪ/
daughter	don't	doubt	dance	during	die
dog	door	down			

Everyday Language

Phrases	*Sentences*
/dɪ/	
1. good condition	1. It's in good condition.
2. is dinner ready	2. What time is dinner ready?
3. did you	3. Did you hear the news?
4. dear _____	4. Dear _____, we miss you.
5. a distance	5. That's quite a distance.
/de/	
1. daily paper	1. We get a daily paper.
2. have a date	2. Do you have a date?
3. take one day	3. Just take one day at a time.
4. today is	4. Today is the first day.
5. face danger	5. He faces danger every day.

Phrases	*Sentences*
/di/	
1. big deal	1. That's no big deal.
2. pretty deep	2. It's in pretty deep.
3. good idea	3. That's a good idea.
4. indeed I	4. Indeed I will!
5. you deal	5. It's your deal.
/du/	
1. do you	1. What do you do?
2. sworn duty	2. It's his sworn duty.
3. they'll produce	3. They'll producc the evidence.
4. past due	4. Your book is past due.
5. what to do	5. Do you know what to do?
/dʌ/	
1. does it	1. Does it hurt much?
2. really doesn't	2. No, it really doesn't.
3. nearly done	3. I'm nearly done.
4. that's double	4. That's double the amount.
5. doesn't matter	5. It doesn't matter now.
/dɛ/	
1. wouldn't dare	1. You wouldn't dare!
2. I dare	2. I dare you!
3. is dead	3. My flower is dead.
4. it's death	4. It's death is a blessing.
5. how dare you	5. How dare you say that!
/da/	
1. got dark	1. It got dark early.
2. call the doctor	2. Call the doctor, quick!
3. another dollar	3. You'll need another dollar.
4. dollar a day	4. A dollar a day isn't much.
5. in the dark	5. Can you see in the dark?
/dɔ/	
1. my daughter	1. My daughter is home.
2. like my dog	2. Do you like my dog?
3. your daughter	3. Your daughter called me.
4. dog sleep	4. Where does your dog sleep?
5. feed your dog	5. What do you feed your dog?

Phrases	*Sentences*
/do/	
1. don't say	1. Don't say that again.
2. lock the door	2. Did you lock the door?
3. hold the door	3. Hold the door for me.
4. I don't	4. I don't have time.
5. don't care	5. You just don't care.
/daʊ/	
1. I doubt	1. I doubt if he comes.
2. come down	2. Come down when you finish.
3. doubt about it	3. There's no doubt about it!
4. down the hall	4. She lives down the hall.
5. to doubt you	5. You cause me to doubt you.
/dæ/	
1. dance fast	1. Can you dance fast?
2. like to dance	2. Would you like to dance?
3. the dance	3. The dance is at nine.
4. to the dance	4. Want to go to the dance?
5. you dance	5. You dance very well.
/dɝ/	
1. during lunch	1. We can talk during lunch.
2. during rush hour	2. Traffic is bad during rush hour.
3. during the week	3. During the week I can't.
4. during the day	4. There's little time during the day.
5. during class	5. We'll finish during class.
/daɪ/	
1. just die	1. Couldn't you just die!
2. they'll die	2. They'll die without water.
3. she die	3. Will she die, doctor?
4. people die	4. People die every day.
5. many people die	5. Too many people die in accidents.

/d/ CONTEXTS

Distinctive features: linguaalveolar, plosive, voiced
/d/ ***vowel combinations:*** Initial position of an unstressed syllable

Deep Test

/dɪ/ decide /dɛ/ president /do/ window /dɚ/ under /də/ industry

Common Words

/dɪ/	/dɚ/	/də/	/dɛ/	/do/
already	order	industry	president	window
decide	shoulder			
declare	under			
degree	understand			
demand	wonder			
department	wonderful			
desire				
destroy				
direct				
direction				
discover				
divide				
garden				
golden				
lady				
study				

Everyday Language

Phrases	*Sentences*
/dɪ/	
1. have to decide	1. You'll just have to decide.
2. what department	2. What department is this?
3. let's divide	3. Let's divide the winnings.
4. no desire	4. I've no desire to go.
5. they'll demand	5. They'll demand cash.
/dɚ/	
1. your order	1. May I take your order?
2. shoulder hurts	2. My shoulder hurts.
3. I wonder	3. I wonder what happened?
4. understand anything	4. Can't you understand anything?
5. look under	5. Look under the sofa.
/də/	
1. lots of industry	1. There's lots of industry there.
2. new industry	2. This is a new industry.
3. in industry	3. He works in industry.
4. for industry	4. They use it for industry.
5. depends on industry	5. The economy depends on industry.

Phrases	*Sentences*
/dɛ/	
1. new president	1. Who's the new president?
2. run for president	2. She'll run for president.
3. president-elect now	3. He's president-elect now.
4. of the president	4. This is the office of the president.
5. nominations for president	5. Are there any nominations for president?
/do/	
1. another window	1. We need another window.
2. open the window	2. Open the window, please.
3. close the window	3. Close the window, please.
4. broke the window	4. Who broke the window?
5. out the window	5. It went out the window.

/d/ CONTEXTS

Distinctive features: linguaalveolar, plosive, voiced
/d/ ***vowel combinations:*** Final position of a stressed syllable

Deep Test

/id/ need	/ɛd/ bed	/od/ road	/ɝd/ word	/aɪd/ side
/ɪd/ did	/æd/ add	/ʊd/ good	/ʌd/ sudden	/aʊd/ cloud
/ed/ paid	/ɑd/ god	/ud/ food		

Common Words

/ɛd/	/aɪd/	/ed/	/ʊd/	/id/	/æd/	/ɝd/
bed	beside	afraid	could	indeed	add	bird
dead	decide	laid	good	lead	bad	heard
head	divide	made	should	leader	glad	third
instead	guide	paid	stood	need	had	word
led	I'd	shade	wood			
read	outside	trade	would			
ready	provide					
red	ride					
said	side					
spread	tried					

/ʌd/	/ɪd/	/ɑd/	/aʊd/	/ud/	/od/
blood	consider	god	cloud	food	road
sudden	did	modern	crowd	include	
suddenly	middle				

Everyday Language

Phrases	*Sentences*
/ɛd/	
1. in bed	1. She's still in bed.
2. your head	2. Use your head this time.
3. have you read	3. Have you read that book?
4. the red one	4. Wear the red one.
5. doesn't spread	5. I hope it doesn't spread.
/aɪd/	
1. I'd like	1. I'd like some more.
2. outside now	2. Take it outside now.
3. short ride	3. That's a short ride.
4. we tried	4. We tried to help them.
5. on its side	5. Turn it on its side.
/ed/	
1. I'm afraid	1. I'm afraid its over.
2. laid an egg	2. They really laid an egg!
3. who made	3. Who made that remark?
4. she'll trade	4. She'll trade you even.
5. made certain	5. We've made certain of it.
/ʊd/	
1. should that	1. Should that be there?
2. good luck	2. Good luck to you!
3. stood still	3. He just stood still.
4. would be	4. It would be better.
5. should go	5. Someone should go in.
/id/	
1. you lead	1. You lead, I'll follow.
2. follow the leader	2. Sounds like "Follow the Leader."
3. you need	3. You need some help.
4. indeed I	4. Indeed, I do need something.
5. lead anywhere	5. That doesn't lead anywhere.
/æd/	
1. just add	1. Just add it to my bill.
2. a bad break	2. That's a bad break.
3. I'm glad	3. I'm glad you're here.
4. we had	4. We had a ball!
5. add mine	5. Add mine to the list.

Phrases	*Sentences*
/ɝd/	
1. a black bird	1. Is that a black bird?
2. I heard	2. I heard a cute story.
3. the third time	3. That's the third time.
4. my word	4. My word, that's nice!
5. keep his word	5. He'll keep his word.
/ʌd/	
1. see blood	1. He can't stand to see blood.
2. sudden death	2. Sudden death wins!
3. sudden move	3. Any sudden move could break it.
4. suddenly it	4. Suddenly it was all over.
5. my blood	5. My blood ran cold!
/ɪd/	
1. consider it	1. Did you consider it?
2. in the middle	2. She'll be in the middle.
3. did well	3. You did well this time.
4. consider it	4. I consider it settled.
5. caught in the middle	5. Don't get caught in the middle.
/ɑd/	
1. modern look	1. That's a modern look.
2. for a god	2. It's fit for a god.
3. like a god	3. He acts like a god.
4. modern dance	4. Modern dance is fun.
5. modern house	5. Is it a modern house?
/aʊd/	
1. not a cloud	1. Not a cloud in the sky.
2. at the crowd	2. Just look at the crowd!
3. don't crowd	3. Don't crowd in now!
4. for the cloud	4. Watch for the cloud of smoke.
5. three's a crowd	5. Three's a crowd they say.
/ud/	
1. good food	1. That was good food.
2. include a tip	2. Does that include a tip?
3. my food	3. My food is cold!
4. include them	4. Include them in the group.
5. include enough	5. Include enough return postage.

Phrases	*Sentences*
/od/	
1. the next road	1. Turn on the next road.
2. long road	2. It's a long road ahead.
3. on this road	3. They live on this road.
4. the second road	4. Stop at the second road.
5. this road	5. This road is blocked.

/d/ CONTEXTS

Distinctive features: linguaalveolar, plosive, voiced
/d/ ***vowel combinations:*** Final position of an unstressed syllable

Deep Test

/ɪd/ hundred /æd/ admit /od/ railroad /ɚd/ forward /əd/ method

Comm Words

/əd/	/æd/	/ɚd/	/ɪd/	/od/
method	admit	forward	hundred	railroad
period	advance	record		
thousand				

Everyday Language

Phrases	*Sentences*
/əd/	
1. a new method	1. Is that a new method?
2. he said period	2. That's what he said, period.
3. next period	3. Next period will go fast.
4. had a thousand	4. Wish I had a thousand!
5. either method	5. Either method will work.
/æd/	
1. I admit	1. I admit my faults.
2. have an advance	2. May I have an advance?
3. didn't advance	3. They didn't advance far.
4. admit it	4. Did he admit it?
5. admit anything	5. He won't admit anything.

Phrases	*Sentences*
/ɚd/	
1. very forward	1. She's very forward.
2. my record	2. Want to hear my record?
3. new record	3. They have out a new record.
4. move it forward	4. Move it forward an inch.
5. far forward	5. It's too far forward now.
/ɪd/	
1. hundred times	1. Write it a hundred times.
2. two hundred	2. It cost two hundred dollars.
3. over a hundred	3. His temperature is over a hundred!
4. a hundred more	4. A hundred more came today.
5. below a hundred	5. It's below a hundred now.
/od/	
1. railroad crossing	1. Watch the railroad crossing.
2. railroad work	2. Railroad work is hard.
3. railroad has	3. The railroad has an exciting history.
4. railroad station	4. We'll meet at the railroad station.
5. what railroad	5. What railroad is that?

/k/ CONTEXTS

Distinctive features: linguavelar, plosive, voiceless
/k/ ***vowel combinations:*** Initial position of a stressed syllable

Deep Test

/ki/ keep	/kɛ/ care	/kɔ/ call	/ku/ cool	/kaɪ/ kind
/kɪ/ kiss	/kæ/ can	/ko/ coat	/kʌ/ come	/kaʊ/ count
/ke/ came	/kɑ/ car	/kʊ/ could		

Common Words

/kʌ/	/ko/	/kɔ/	/kɛ/	/kæ/	/kɑ/
become	coal	call	care	camp	car
color	coat	caught	carry	can	college
come	cold	cause	character	captain	common
coming	course	cost	kept	catch	cotton
company	count	corner			
country					
cover					
cup					
cut					
discover					

/kɪ/	/ke/	/ki/	/kʊ/	/ku/	/kaɪ/	/kaʊ/
kill	became	keep	could	cool	kind	count
king	came					
kiss	case					
kitchen						

Everyday Language

Phrases	*Sentences*
/kʌ/	
1. become of us	1. What will become of us?
2. new color	2. That's a new color.
3. having company	3. We're having company tonight.
4. the cover	4. Close the cover tightly.
5. cup of coffee	5. Want a cup of coffee?
/ko/	
1. as coal	1. It's as black as coal.
2. cold enough	2. Keep it cold enough.
3. my coat	3. You can wear my coat.
4. of course	4. Of course you can.
5. to court	5. They'll take him to court.
/kɔ/	
1. he'll call	1. He'll call later tonight.
2. caught him	2. They caught him red-handed.
3. won't cost	3. It won't cost that much.
4. good cause	4. It's for a good cause.
5. call me	5. Call me when you can.

Phrases	*Sentences*
/kɛ/	
1. don't care	1. I just don't care anymore.
2. main character	2. Who's the main character?
3. she kept	3. She kept her word.
4. carry that	4. You can carry that.
5. lot of care	5. It takes a lot of care.
/kæ/	
1. camp is	1. Camp is just over the hill.
2. I can	2. I can if he can.
3. catch a cold	3. He couldn't catch a cold!
4. the captain	4. Listen, the captain is speaking.
5. we can	5. We can hear you now.
/kɑ/	
1. new car	1. Is that a new car?
2. what college	2. What college is he in?
3. common sense	3. Use your common sense.
4. cotton is king	4. Cotton is king, they say.
5. have the car	5. May I have the car tonight?
/kɪ/	
1. kill yourself	1. Don't kill yourself!
2. like a king	2. I feel like a king.
3. kiss me	3. Kiss me, you fool!
4. the kitchen	4. My favorite room is the kitchen.
5. in the kitchen	5. We spend time in the kitchen, too.
/ke/	
1. it became	1. It became too much.
2. he came	2. He came right over.
3. whole case	3. Let's get a whole case.
4. case comes up	4. The case comes up Tuesday.
5. whatever became	5. Whatever became of her?
/ki/	
1. can't keep	1. You can't keep a good man down.
2. keep it	2. Where should we keep it?
3. keep talking	3. Keep talking, I'm listening.
4. keep it up	4. Keep it up and you're fired!
5. keep up	5. Keep up the good work!

Phrases	*Sentences*
/kʊ/	
1. he could	1. He could if he would.
2. could you	2. Could you help out?
3. how could	3. Oh, how could you!
4. I could	4. I could tell you a lot.
5. could finish	5. We could finish soon.
/ku/	
1. your cool	1. Keep your cool!
2. served cool	2. It's best served cool.
3. cool reception	3. That was a cool reception.
4. windy and cool	4. Today will be windy and cool.
5. cool off	5. Why don't you cool off?
/kaɪ/	
1. what kind	1. What kind is it?
2. my kind	2. He isn't my kind.
3. be kind	3. Be kind to animals.
4. I kind	4. I kind of like her.
5. another kind	5. Another kind will do.
/kaʊ/	
1. don't count	1. Don't count me out!
2. count them	2. Count them again.
3. count on it	3. You can't count on it.
4. close count	4. Keep a close count.
5. Count Dracula	5. Who was Count Dracula?

/k/ **CONTEXTS**

Distinctive features: linguavelar, plosive, voiceless
/k/ ***vowel combinations:*** Initial position of an unstressed syllable

Deep Test

/kɪ/ market   /kə/ command

Common Words

/kə/	/kɪ/
command	market
complete	
condition	
consider	
contain	
continue	
control	

Everyday Language

Phrases	*Sentences*
/kə/	
1. I command	1. I command you to stop!
2. be complete	2. It won't be complete without you.
3. one condition	3. He'll do it on one condition.
4. continue reading	4. Let's continue reading.
5. lost control	5. I think we've lost control.
/kɪ/	
1. no market	1. There's no market for it.
2. to the market	2. Should we go to the market?
3. market basket	3. We'll need a market basket?
4. stock market	4. Do you play the stock market?
5. nearest market	5. Where's the nearest market?

/k/ CONTEXTS

Distinctive features: linguavelar, plosive, voiceless
/k/ ***vowel combinations:*** Final position of a stressed syllable

Deep Test

/ik/ week	/ɛk/ neck	/ɑk/ doctor	/ok/ broken	/ɝk/work
/ɪk/ pick	/æk/ action	/ɔk/ walk	/ʊk/ took	/aɪk/ like
/ek/ take				

Common Words

/ɪk/	/ek/	/ɛk/	/æk/	/ʊk/	/ik/	/ɑk/
pick	break	check	action	book	seek	doctor
picture	lake	direction	back	cook	speak	rock
quickly	make	exercise	black	look	week	stock
sick	take	neck	practice	took		
stick	taken					

/ok/	/ɔk/	/ɝk/	/aɪk/
broken	talk	work	like
smoke	walk		

Everyday Language

Phrases	*Sentences*
/ɪk/	
1. try to pick	1. Try to pick a good one.
2. a good picture	2. Isn't that a good picture?
3. run quickly	3. Run quickly and tell them!
4. makes me sick	4. That just makes me sick!
5. carry a big stick	5. Who said, "Carry a big stick"?
/ek/	
1. break it	1. Break it to him gently.
2. to the lake	2. A trip to the lake would be great.
3. Don't make	3. Don't make me laugh!
4. I've taken	4. I've taken about all I can.
5. take this	5. You take this and I'll take that.
/ɛk/	
1. write a check	1. Just write a check.
2. which direction	2. Which direction is it?
3. more exercise	3. You need more exercise.
4. neck out	4. Don't stick your neck out.
5. check on	5. I'll check on it.
/æk/	
1. some action	1. Let's get some action!
2. right back	2. I'll be right back.
3. practice makes	3. Remember practice makes perfect.
4. the black one	4. The black one is my favorite.
5. turned his back	5. He just turned his back on us.

Phrases	*Sentences*
/ʊk/	
1. a new book	1. He's written a new book.
2. great cook	2. She's a great cook.
3. look here	3. Look here–I didn't do it!
4. took our time	4. We just took our time.
5. the cook book	5. Where's the cook book?
/ik/	
1. seek his fortune	1. He went to seek his fortune.
2. who'll speak	2. Who'll speak to that point?
3. a week from	3. We'll meet a week from today.
4. Hide'n Seek	4. The kids are playing Hide'n Seek.
5. whole week	5. A whole week has gone by.
/ɑk/	
1. need a doctor	1. We need a doctor here.
2. rock the boat	2. Don't rock the boat.
3. stock up	3. Better stock up on that.
4. your doctor	4. Who's your doctor?
5. as a rock	5. It's hard as a rock.
/ok/	
1. isn't broken	1. I hope it isn't broken.
2. smell smoke	2. Do you smell smoke?
3. you spoke	3. You spoke too soon.
4. he's broken	4. He's broken his promise.
5. smoke cigars	5. Do you smoke cigars?
/ɔk/	
1. you talk	1. You talk too much.
2. for a walk	2. Let's go for a walk.
3. I'll walk	3. It isn't far, so I'll walk.
4. long walk	4. A long walk is good exercise.
5. have a talk	5. We need to have a talk.
/ɝk/	
1. it will work	1. Do you think it will work?
2. all work	2. All work and no play . . .
3. do you work	3. Where do you work?
4. work it out	4. We can work it out!
5. go to work	5. Time to go to work!

Phrases	*Sentences*
/aɪk/	
1. don't like it	1. I don't like it a bit.
2. like it or not	2. Like it or not, we must.
3. looks like	3. It looks like rain.
4. kind of like	4. It's kind of like ice cream.
5. you like it	5. If you like it, tell her.

/k/ CONTEXTS

Distinctive features: linguavelar, plosive, voiceless
/k/ ***vowel combinations:*** Final position of an unstressed syllable

Deep Test

/ɪk/ music /ɛk/ except /æk/ accept /ək/ success

Common Words

/ɛk/	/ɪk/	/æk/	/ək/
except	character	accept	success
expect	music		
experience	public		
explain			
express			

Everyday Language

Phrases	*Sentences*
/ɛk/	
1. can you expect	1. What can you expect?
2. my experience	2. That's not my experience.
3. explain yourself	3. Well, explain yourself.
4. can't express	4. I just can't express how I feel.
5. except for you	5. Except for you, I'd quit.
/ɪk/	
1. that's music	1. That's music to my ears!
2. public figure	2. He's a powerful public figure.
3. that character	3. Who's that character?
4. her music	4. You'll love her music.
5. public servant	5. Want to be a public servant?

Phrases	*Sentences*
/æk/	
1. accept it	1. I can't accept it.
2. accept the award	2. Who'll accept the award?
3. accept your fate	3. Accept your fate gracefully.
4. accept you	4. Don't worry, they'll accept you.
5. accept my apology	5. Will you accept my apology?
/ək/	
1. have success	1. I hope you have success.
2. your success	2. What's the secret of your success?
3. success comes	3. Success comes in can's.
4. her success	4. Her success is remarkable.
5. to success	5. We'll, here's to success!

/k/ **CONTEXTS**

Distinctive features: linguavelar, plosive, voiceless
/k/ ***blends:*** Initial position of a stressed syllable

Deep Test

/kw/ queen /kl/ clean

Common Words

/kl/	/kw/
claim	quarter
class	queen
clean	question
clear	quickly
close	quite
clothes	require
cloud	
club	
declare	
include	

Everyday Language

Phrases	*Sentences*
/kl/	
1. no claim	1. You have no claim.
2. what class	2. What class are you in?
3. clear enough	3. It's clear enough to me.
4. my clothes	4. My clothes are a mess!
5. clean it	5. Well, clean it up!
/kw/	
1. a quarter	1. Loan me a quarter.
2. she's queen	2. She's "queen for a day."
3. quite right	3. You're quite right.
4. did it quickly	4. They did it quickly.
5. no question	5. There's no question about it.

/k/ CONTEXTS

Distinctive features: linguavelar, plosive, voiceless
/k/ ***blends:*** Final position of a stressed syllable

Deep Test

/kt/ act /ks/ box /kst/ next

Common Words

/kt/	/ks/	/kst/
act	box	next
direct	six	
expect		
fact		
object		

Everyday Language

Phrases	*Sentences*
/kt/	
1. act dumb	1. Don't act dumb!
2. very direct	2. He's very direct, isn't he?
3. known fact	3. That's a known fact.
4. I expect	4. I expect only the best.
5. do you object	5. Why do you object?
/ks/	
1. where's the box.	1. Where's the box it came in?
2. box it up	2. Just box it up for me.
3. six will	3. Six will be plenty.
4. small box	4. It's just a small box.
5. six of one	5. Six of one, half dozen ____.
/kst/	
1. next time	1. Next time you drive.
2. be next	2. Want to be next?
3. next door	3. He's just next door.
4. next week	4. Next week we go home.
5. next to me	5. He works next to me.

/k/ CONTEXTS

Distinctive features: linguavelar, plosive, voiceless
/k/ ***blends:*** Final position of an unstressed syllable

Deep Test

/kt/ subject

Common Words

/kt/
subject

Everyday Language

Phrases	*Sentences*
/kt/	
1. dumb subject	1. This is a dumb subject.
2. this subject	2. This subject bores me.
3. main subject	3. What's the main subject?
4. one subject	4. Here's one subject you'll like–money!
5. she's subject	5. She's subject to colds.

/g/ CONTEXTS

Distinctive features: linguavelar, plosive, voiced
/g/ *vowel combinations:* Initial position of a stressed syllable

Deep Test

/gɪ/ give	/gɛ/ get	/gɑ/ got	/go/ ago	/gʌ/ government
/ge/ gave	/gæ/ began	/gɔ/ gone	/gɝ/ girl	/gaɪ/ guide

Common Words

/gɛ/	/gɑ/	/ge/	/go/	/gɪ/	/gæ/	/gɔ/
again	garden	gain	ago	begin	began	gone
against	god	game	going	give	gather	
forget	got	gate	gold	given	gather	
get	guard	gave	golden			
guess	regard					
together						

/gɝ/	/gə/	/gaɪ/
girl	government	guide

Everyday Language

Phrases	*Sentences*
/gɛ/	
1. did it again	1. Well, they did it again!
2. against it	2. I'm not against it, but . . .
3. don't forget	3. Don't forget to write.
4. go together	4. Let's all go together.
5. a wild guess	5. It's just a wild guess.

Phrases	*Sentences*
/ga/	
1. a bigger garden	1. Just plant a bigger garden.
2. he's a god	2. He thinks he's a god.
3. guard up	3. Keep your guard up!
4. don't regard	4. We don't regard that as important.
5. got it	5. I've got it—we'll have a party!
/ge/	
1. little gain	1. A little gain is OK.
2. playing a game	2. We're just playing a game.
3. gave up	3. She gave up at last.
4. opened the gate	4. Who opened the gate?
5. would you gain	5. What would you gain?
/go/	
1. long ago	1. That was long ago.
2. are you going	2. When are you going?
3. good as gold	3. It's as good as gold.
4. a golden touch	4. She has a golden touch.
5. a minute ago	5. He was here a minute ago.
/gɪ/	
1. where to begin	1. Where to begin is the question.
2. give up	2. Don't give up yet.
3. gives it	3. She gives it a lot of thought.
4. at the front	4. Begin at the front and work back.
5. begin somehow	5. You have to begin somehow.
/gæ/	
1. they began	1. They began late again.
2. I gather	2. I gather they usually do.
3. gather around	3. Gather around for the fun.
4. began long ago	4. It all began long ago.
5. began to rain	5. Suddenly it began to rain.
/gɔ/	
1. all gone	1. Well, it's all gone now.
2. they're gone	2. They're gone for the weekend.
3. gone over it	3. I've gone over it twice.
4. gone too far	4. We've gone too far to stop.
5. long gone	5. I think he's long gone.

Phrases	*Sentences*
/gɝ/	
1. girl friend	1. Who's your girl friend?
2. a nice girl	2. She's really a nice girl.
3. girl talk	3. It sounds like "girl talk."
4. new girl	4. Who's the new girl?
5. only a girl	5. Only a girl would know!
/gə/	
1. a government job	1. Would you like a government job?
2. local government	2. It's up to local government.
3. good government	3. He's for good government.
4. less government	4. What we need is less government.
5. government funds	5. We should try for government funds.
/gaɪ/	
1. guide book	1. Where's the guide book?
2. hire a guide	2. You'll need to hire a guide.
3. guide us	3. Can you guide us?
4. can't guide	4. I can't guide very straight.
5. guide to the left	5. Guide to the left, then right.

/g/ CONTEXTS

Distinctive features: linguavelar, plosive, voiced
/g/ ***vowel combinations:*** Initial position of an unstressed syllable

Deep Test

/gɚ/ finger

Common Words

/gɚ/

finger
sugar

Everyday Language

Phrases	*Sentences*
/gɚ/	
1. sugar cookie	1. That's a sugar cookie.
2. sugar is sweet	2. Sugar is sweet and _____.
3. one finger	3. Hold up one finger.
4. put my finger	4. I can't put my finger on it.
5. with your finger	5. Just point with your finger.

/g/ CONTEXTS

Distinctive features: linguavelar, plosive, voiced
/g/ ***vowel combinations:*** Final position of a stressed syllable

Deep Test

/ɪg/ big /ɛg/ egg /æg/ bag /ɔg/ dog

Common Words

/ɪg/	/ɛg/	/æg/	/ɔg/
big	egg	bag	dog
figure	leg		

Everyday Language

Phrases	*Sentences*
/ɪg/	
1. big surprise	1. You're in for a big surprise.
2. I figure	2. I figure I can take it.
3. fine figure	3. You cut a fine figure.
4. figure it out	4. You'll just have to figure it out.
5. great figure	5. She has a great figure.
/ɛg/	
1. one egg	1. It takes only one egg.
2. egg him on	2. They tried to "egg him on."
3. my leg	3. You're pulling my leg.
4. boiled egg	4. I'll have a boiled egg.
5. on one leg	5. Stand on one leg, please.

Phrases

/æg/

1. in the bag
2. my bag
3. put your bag
4. another bag
5. one bag

Sentences

1. It's in the bag.
2. Who took my bag?
3. Put your bag down here.
4. We'll need another bag.
5. One bag is plenty.

Phrases

/ɔg/

1. have a dog
2. it's a dog
3. whose dog
4. doggone
5. like a dog

Sentences

1. Do you have a dog?
2. I think its a dog.
3. Whose dog is that?
4. I'll be doggone!
5. He works like a dog.

/g/ CONTEXTS

Distinctive features: linguavelar, plosive, voiced
/g/ ***vowel combinations:*** Final position of an unstressed syllable

Deep Test

/ɛg/ example /əg/ suggest

Common Words

/ɛg/	/dg/
example	suggest

Everyday Language

Phrases

/ɛg/

1. for example
2. good example
3. an example
4. one example
5. bad example

Sentences

1. For example, here's one.
2. Give me one good example.
3. Set an example for others.
4. One example will do.
5. That's a bad example.

Phrases	*Sentences*
/əg/	
1. would you suggest	1. What would you suggest?
2. I suggest	2. I suggest a rest.
3. suggest that	3. You would suggest that!
4. suggest more	4. It's crazy to suggest more.
5. we'll suggest	5. We'll suggest it to the boss.

/g/ CONTEXTS

Distinctive features: linguavelar, plosive, voiced
/g/ ***blends:*** Initial position of a stressed syllable

Deep Test

/gr/ grow   /gl/ glad

Common Words

/gr/	/gl/
agree	glad
degree	glass
grant	
grass	
gray	
great	
green	
grew	
ground	
group	
grow	

Everyday Language

Phrases	*Sentences*
/gr/	
1. great day	1. It's a great day!
2. grow up	2. Why don't you grow up?
3. paint it green	3. Paint it green or white.
4. cut the grass	4. I hate to cut the grass.
5. I agree	5. I agree, she's beautiful!

Phrases	*Sentences*
/gl/	
1. I'm glad	1. I'm glad you're here.
2. fill your glass	2. Let me fill your glass.
3. no more glad	3. You're no more glad than I!
4. my glass	4. Is this my glass?
5. in glass houses	5. People in glass houses _____.

/f/ CONTEXTS

Distinctive features: labiodental, fricative-continuant, voiceless
/f/ ***vowel combinations:*** Initial position of a stressed syllable

Deep Test

/fi/ feel	/fɛ/ fell	/fɑ/ far	/fo/ four	/fu/ food	/faɪ/ five
/fɪ/ fear	/fæ/ fat	/fɔ/ fall	/fʊ/ full	/fɝ/ first	/faʊ/ found
/fe/ face					

Common Words

/fɪ/	/fɔ/	/fɑ/	/fɛ/	/faɪ/	/fæ/	/fe/
fear	fall	far	affair	fight	fact	face
fifty	for	farm	fair	find	family	fail
figure	foreign	farmer	fell	fine	fast	famous
fill	forest	father	fellow	fire	fat	favor
finger	form	follow	felt	five		
finish	former	following				
fit	forward					
fish						

/fo/	/fi/	/fu/	/fʊ/	/fɝ/	/faʊ/
before	feel	food	foot	first	found
force	feet	fool	full	further	
forth	field				
four					

Everyday Language

Phrases	*Sentences*
/fɪ/	
1. never fear	1. Never fear, _____ is here!
2. fill it	2. Fill it with regular, please.
3. caught the fish	3. Who caught the fish?
4. finish soon	4. Will you finish soon?
5. your finger	5. Hold up your finger.
/fɔ/	
1. nasty fall	1. That was a nasty fall.
2. who's for	2. Who's for playing tennis?
3. all foreign	3. It's all foreign to me.
4. former director	4. He's the former director.
5. good form	5. That's really good form.
/fɑ/	
1. get far	1. They won't get far.
2. your father	2. Is your father a lawyer?
3. just follow	3. Just follow the directions.
4. their farm	4. Their farm is near here.
5. following close	5. They're following close behind.
/fɛ/	
1. my affair	1. It's not my affair.
2. fair weather	2. Fair weather is forecast.
3. that fellow	3. Who's that fellow?
4. felt fine	4. I felt fine this morning.
5. grades fell	5. My grades fell this term.
/faɪ/	
1. a tough fight	1. It's been a tough fight.
2. find it	2. Did you find it?
3. be fine	3. He'll be fine tomorrow.
4. five times	4. Write each one five times.
5. fire with fire	5. Fight fire with fire.
/fæ/	
1. your family	1. How large is your family?
2. it's a fact	2. It's a fact–it's over.
3. fast work	3. That's pretty fast work!
4. fat raise	4. He got a fat raise.
5. a fact	5. Is that a fact!

Phrases	*Sentences*
/fe/	
1. tend to favor	1. I tend to favor spending.
2. you can fail	2. There's no way you can fail.
3. face him	3. How will I face him?
4. she's famous	4. She's famous for her cakes.
5. if we fail	5. If we fail, we'll try again.
/fo/	
1. before you start	1. Before you start, sit down.
2. force won't help	2. Force won't help this time.
3. come forth	3. Come forth and testify!
4. four more	4. Now there are four more.
5. before I knew	5. It happened before I knew it.
/fi/	
1. feel funny	1. I feel funny today.
2. feet hurt	2. My feet hurt.
3. left field	3. He plays left field.
4. feel we should	4. Do you feel we should?
5. two feet	5. It's two feet too long.
/fʊ/	
1. I'm full	1. No more, I'm full.
2. full day's work	2. It'll be a full day's work.
3. his foot	3. He put his foot in his mouth!
4. about a foot	4. Move it over about a foot.
5. full tank	5. You have a full tank.
/fu/	
1. too much food	1. We've had too much food.
2. fool me	2. You can't fool me.
3. no fool	3. One thing, he's no fool!
4. an old fool	4. There's no fool like an old fool!
5. good fool	5. You can't beat good food.
/fɝ/	
1. try first	1. You'll have to try first.
2. first thing	2. First thing to do is be there.
3. further notice	3. Wait 'til further notice.
4. further news	4. There's been no further news.
5. first place	5. Now we're in first place.

Phrases	*Sentences*
/faʊ/	
1. I found it out	1. I found it out today.
2. was it found	2. Where was it found?
3. found one	3. We only found one.
4. finally found	4. She finally found her match.
5. found the way	5. We found the way after all.

/f/ CONTEXTS

Distinctive features: labiodental, fricative-continuant, voiceless
/f/ ***vowel combinations:*** Initial position of an unstressed syllable

Deep Test

/fɔ/ forget   /fo/ therefore   /fə/ beautiful

Common Words

/fə/	/fɔ/	/fo/
beautiful	forget	therefore
wonderful		

Everyday Language

Phrases	*Sentences*
/fə/	
1. just wonderful	1. I think it's just wonderful!
2. wonderful weather	2. Wonderful weather we're having!
3. beautiful sight	3. That's a beautiful sight.
4. beautiful day	4. Beautiful day for sailing!
5. wonderful teacher	5. She's a wonderful teacher.
/fɔ/	
1. forget to write	1. Don't forget to write.
2. forget to vote	2. Don't forget to vote.
3. forget to ask	3. Don't forget to ask.
4. forget it	4. Forget it—I'll do it!
5. if you forget	5. If you forget, I'll be angry.

Phrases	*Sentences*
/fo/	
1. therefore I am	1. He is; therefore I am.
2. therefore I'm going	2. It's late; therefore I'm going.
3. therefore who	3. Therefore, who can say?
4. therefore they	4. Therefore they both came.
5. therefore tell	5. He's OK; therefore tell him.

/f/ CONTEXTS

Distinctive features: labiodental, fricative-continuant, voiceless
/f/ ***vowel combinations:*** Final position of a stressed syllable

Deep Test

/æf/ after

Common Words

/æf/

after

Everyday Language

Phrases	*Sentences*
/æf/	
1. after you're gone	1. After you're gone, we'll talk.
2. it's after	2. It's after my bedtime.
3. after class	3. See you after class.
4. after the game	4. We'll meet after the game.
5. after you did	5. We got home after you did.

/f/ CONTEXTS

Distinctive features: labiodental, fricative-continuant, voiceless
/f/ ***vowel combinations:*** Final position of an unstressed syllable

Deep Test

/æf/ afternoon

Common Words

/æf/

afternoon

Everyday Language

Phrases	*Sentences*
/æf/	
1. this afternoon	1. See you later this afternoon.
2. afternoon movie	2. Let's watch the afternoon movie.
3. starts this afternoon	3. It starts this afternoon at one.
4. afternoon nap	4. I miss my afternoon nap.
5. afternoon will be	5. This afternoon will be better.

/f/ CONTEXTS

Distinctive features: labiodental, fricative-continuant, voiceless
/f/ ***blends:*** Initial position of a stressed syllable

Deep Test

/fl/ floor /fr/ free

Common Words

/fr/	/fl/
afraid	floor
free	flow
fresh	flower
friend	fly
from	
front	
fruit	

Everyday Language

Phrases / *Sentences*

/fr/

Phrases	Sentences
1. one free	1. Buy one—get one free.
2. good friend	2. He's my good friend.
3. fresh start	3. He'll get a fresh start today.
4. from home	4. Oh boy, a note from home!
5. up front	5. It's what's up front that counts.

/fl/

Phrases	Sentences
1. waxed the floor	1. They just waxed the floor.
2. fly over	2. Will you fly over?
3. flow freely	3. Let it flow freely.
4. flower came	4. A flower came for you.
5. sit on the floor	5. We'll just sit on the floor.

/f/ CONTEXTS

Distinctive features: labiodental, fricative-continuant, voiceless
/f/ ***blends:*** Final position of a stressed syllable

Deep Test

/ft/ left

Common Words

/ft/
left
lift
soft

Everyday Language

/ft/

Phrases	Sentences
1. he left	1. He left a note.
2. lift me up	2. Lift me up so I can see.
3. really soft	3. It's really soft to touch.
4. a soft touch	4. You're a soft touch, you know.
5. to the left	5. Turn it to the left.

/v/ CONTEXTS

Distinctive features: labiodental, fricative-continuant, voiced
/v/ ***vowel combinations:*** Initial position of a stressed syllable

Deep Test

/vɪ/ visit	/væ/ advance	/vaɪ/ divide	/vɔɪ/ voice	/vju/ view
/vɛ/ very	/vo/ vote			

Common Words

/væ/	/vɪ/	/vɛ/	/vaɪ/	/vɔɪ/	/vju/	/vo/
advance	village	various	divide	voice	view	vote
valley	visit	very	provide			
value						

Everyday Language

Phrases	*Sentences*
/væ/	
1. advance in	1. I'll need an advance in pay.
2. in the valley	2. They live in the valley.
3. down in the valley	3. Let's sing "Down in the Valley."
4. good value	4. That's a good value.
5. chance to advance	5. There's a good chance to advance.
/vɪ/	
1. village mayor	1. He's the village mayor.
2. come visit	2. Come visit us soon.
3. visit the capitol	3. Did you visit the capitol?
4. to the village	4. We moved to the village.
5. brief visit	5. We had a brief visit.
/vɛ/	
1. various ways	1. There are various ways.
2. very much	2. Thank you very much.
3. very tired	3. I'm very tired tonight.
4. various people	4. Various people could do it.
5. very cold	5. It'll be very cold tonight.

Phrases	*Sentences*
/vaɪ/	
1. have to divide	1. First you have to divide.
2. we'll provide	2. We'll provide the salad.
3. divide the property	3. How did they divide the property?
4. they'll provide	4. They'll provide a room.
5. you divide it	5. You divide it into thirds.
/vɔɪ/	
1. your voice	1. Your voice sounds terrible.
2. voice training	2. Are you in voice training?
3. voice your opinion	3. Voice your opinion soon!
4. voice teacher	4. He's a voice teacher.
5. her voice	5. I recognized her voice.
/vju/	
1. great view	1. It's a great view!
2. point of view	2. That's one point of view.
3. view it	3. I view it as serious.
4. let's view	4. Let's view the film first.
5. my view	5. My view is different.
/vo/	
1. tie vote	1. There was a tie vote.
2. you vote	2. Did you vote yet?
3. my vote	3. You get my vote.
4. let's vote	4. Let's vote on it.
5. vote no	5. I vote "No."

/v/ CONTEXTS

Distinctive features: labiodental, fricative-continuant, voiced
/v/ ***vowel combinations:*** Initial position of an unstressed syllable

Deep Test

/vɚ/over /vɪ/ even

Common Words

/vɚ/	/vɪ/
ever	even
every	service
everything	
favor	
heaven	
heavy	
never	
over	
seven	
several	
silver	
whatever	

Everyday Language

Phrases	*Sentences*
/vɚ/	
1. a favor	1. Do me a favor.
2. finally over	2. It's finally over
3. with silver	3. Cross my palm with silver.
4. I never	4. I never could do that.
5. over there	5. Put it over there.
/vɪ/	
1. even know	1. I don't even know him.
2. good service	2. They give good service.
3. service for eight	3. We'll need service for eight.
4. get them even	4. Try to get them even.
5. room service	5. Let's call room service.

/v/ CONTEXTS

Distinctive features: labiodental, fricative-continuant, voiced
/v/ ***vowel combinations:*** Final position of a stressed syllable

Deep Test

/ɪv/ give /æv/ have /uv/ move /ɝv/ serve /ʌv/ above /aɪv/ five
/ev/ gave

Common Words

/iv/	/ɪv/	/uv/	/ʌv/	/ev/	/aɪv/	/æv/	/ɝv/
believe	give	move	above	gave	arrive	have	serve
evening	given	movement	love	save	drive	travel	
leave	live	prove	of	wave	five		
receive	river	remove					

Everyday Language

Phrases	*Sentences*
/iv/	
1. believe in	1. You have to believe in yourself.
2. evening show	2. The evening show is at eight.
3. leave your coat	3. Did you leave your coat?
4. receive a check	4. We'll receive a check.
5. believe	5. Do you believe that story?
/ɪv/	
1. give it	1. Give it a try!
2. given up	2. You haven't given up?
3. do you live	3. Where do you live?
4. the river	4. The river is high right now.
5. give up	5. I give up!
/uv/	
1. they move	1. Where did they move?
2. much movement	2. There's too much movement.
3. prove it	3. Can they prove it?
4. remove the label	4. To open it, remove the label first.
5. not to move	5. Try not to move.
/ʌv/	
1. above average	1. She's above average.
2. I love	2. I love chocolate.
3. love you	3. I love you.
4. made of	4. What's that made of?
5. love it	5. Oh, you'll love it!
/ev/	
1. gave up	1. They gave up too soon.
2. save your money	2. Save your money for tomorrow.
3. wave as	3. Wave as you go by!
4. who gave	4. Who gave you that?
5. make a wave	5. Don't make a wave!

Phrases	*Sentences*
/aɪv/	
1. we arrive	1. When do we arrive?
2. drive a little	2. Drive a little slower.
3. five times	3. Five times five is ____.
4. arrive early	4. They always arrive early.
5. five dollars	5. You owe me five dollars.
/æv/	
1. you have	1. What'll you have?
2. I travel	2. I travel a lot.
3. have to go	3. We have to go soon.
4. like to travel	4. Do you like to travel?
5. have time	5. Do you have time now?
/ɝv/	
1. your serve	1. It's your serve.
2. help me serve	2. Will you help me serve?
3. serve yourself	3. Just serve yourself.
4. he'll serve	4. He'll serve one term.
5. serve it	5. Serve it hot.

/v/ CONTEXTS

Distinctive features: labiodental, fricative-continuant, voiced
/v/ ***vowel combinations:*** Final position of an unstressed syllable

Deep Test

/ɪv/ native

Common Words

/ɪv/

native

Everyday Language

Phrases	*Sentences*
/ɪv/	
1. native plant	1. Is that a native plant?
2. he's a native	2. He's a native of that country.
3. a native	3. Let's ask a native.
4. native grasses	4. These are native grasses.
5. native food	5. Try the native food.

/θ/ CONTEXTS

Distinctive features: linguadental (interdental), fricative-continuant, voiceless
/θ/ ***vowel combinations:*** Initial position of a stressed syllable

Deep Test

/θɪ/ thin /θæ/ thank /θɔ/ thought /θɝ/ third /θaʊ/ thousand

Common Words

/θɪ/	/θæ/	/θɔ/	/θɝ/	/θaʊ/
thin	thank	thought	third	thousand
thing				
think				

Everyday Language

Phrases	*Sentences*
/θɪ/	
1. too thin	1. You're much too thin.
2. thin slice	2. Just a thin slice for me.
3. he'll think	3. He'll think you're crazy!
4. one thing	4. It's just one thing after another!
5. say a thing	5. I didn't say a thing.
/θæ/	
1. thank you	1. Thank you kindly.
2. thank goodness	2. Thank goodness for that!
3. thank me	3. Don't thank me.
4. thank you enough	4. I just can't thank you enough.
5. thank me	5. You'll thank me later.

Phrases	*Sentences*
/θɔ/	
1. thought so	1. I just thought so.
2. he thought	2. He thought about it.
3. they thought	3. They thought they were smart.
4. a thought	4. Don't give it a thought.
5. good thought	5. That's a good thought.
/θɝ/	
1. third time	1. It's the third time.
2. about a third	2. There's about a third left.
3. one third	3. One third voted "No."
4. third seat	4. Take the third seat over.
5. third to play	5. You'll be third to play.
/θaʊ/	
1. thousand years	1. He'll live a thousand years!
2. thousand miles	2. It's over a thousand miles.
3. twenty thousand	3. There are about twenty thousand people.
4. by the thousand	4. They came by the thousand!
5. a thousand	5. A thousand should do it.

/θ/ CONTEXTS

Distinctive features: linguadental (interdental), fricative-continuant, voiceless
/θ/ vowel combinations: Initial position of an unstressed syllable

Deep Test

/θɪ/ anything

Common Words

/θɪ/

anything
everything
nothing
something

Everyday Language

Phrases	*Sentences*
/θɪ/	
1. anything goes	1. Anything goes, it seems.
2. everything happens	2. Everything happens to me.
3. something seems	3. Something seems wrong here.
4. want anything	4. I don't want anything.
5. something I	5. Something I can do for you?

/θ/ CONTEXTS

Distinctive features: linguadental (interdental), fricative-continuant, voiceless
/θ/ ***vowel combinations:*** Final position of a stressed syllable

Deep Test

/ɛθ/ death /oθ/ both /uθ/ youth /ɝθ/ earth /aʊθ/ mouth
/æθ/ path

Common Words

/ɝθ/	/aʊθ/	/uθ/	/ɛθ/	/oθ/	/æθ/
earth	mouth	truth	death	both	path
worth	south	youth			

Everyday Language

Phrases	*Sentences*
/ɝθ/	
1. what on earth	1. What on earth happened?
2. worth a lot	2. That's worth a lot.
3. he's worth	3. He's worth a million dollars.
4. the earth	4. The earth gets smaller all the time.
5. peace on earth	5. They were singing "Peace on earth . . ."
/aʊθ/	
1. my mouth	1. My mouth is dry.
2. your mouth	2. Just close your mouth!
3. from the south	3. They'll come from the south.
4. in the south	4. The wind is in the south.
5. your mouth	5. Open your mouth wider, please.

Phrases	*Sentences*
/uθ/	
1. plain truth	1. The plain truth is this.
2. tell the truth	2. You must tell the truth.
3. your youth	3. Your youth is gone.
4. regain youth	4. You can't regain youth.
5. the truth	5. The truth will always out!
/ɛθ/	
1. to death	1. You scared me to death!
2. death of me	2. She'll be the death of me!
3. deathbed	3. She's on her deathbed.
4. death doesn't	4. Death doesn't frighten him.
5. slow death	5. It's a slow death.
/oθ/	
1. both of you	1. Both of you come here.
2. both sets	2. We'll need both sets.
3. I both	3. I both love it and hate it.
4. both times	4. We lost both times.
5. both boys	5. Both boys are guilty.
/æθ/	
1. which path	1. Which path do we take?
2. know the path	2. They know the path.
3. build a path	3. We'll build a path.
4. make a path	4. Make a path along here.
5. like a path	5. That looks like a path.

/ð/ CONTEXTS

Distinctive features: linguadental (interdental), fricative-continuant, voiced
/ð/ ***vowel combinations:*** Initial position of a stressed syllable

Deep Test

/ði/ these	/ðe/ they	/ðæ/ that	/ðə/ the
/ðɪ/ this	/ðɛ/ there	/ðo/ those	/ðaʊ/ without

Common Words

/ðɛ/	/ðæ/	/ðo/	/ðɪ/	/ðə/	/ði/	/ðe/	/ðaʊ/
their	than	those	this	the	these	they	without
them	that	though	within				
then							
there							
therefore							

Everyday Language

Phrases	*Sentences*
/ðɛ/	
1. their own way	1. They'll have their own way.
2. there it goes	2. There it goes again.
3. then he	3. Then he just walked away.
4. wasn't there	4. I wasn't there then.
5. one of them	5. One of them told me.
/ðæ/	
1. more than	1. I'm more than happy.
2. that is	2. That is a big help.
3. told you that	3. Who told you that?
4. bigger than	4. I'm bigger than you.
5. smarter than	5. He's smarter than both of us.
/ðo/	
1. those people	1. Those people bore me.
2. refuse though	2. I thought she'd refuse though.
3. though I'm	3. I'll go though I'm scared!
4. are those	4. Are those for sale?
5. those belong	5. Those belong to us.
/ðɪ/	
1. this is	1. This is the end!
2. this time	2. Get it right this time.
3. this was	3. This was the best one.
4. this for	4. Who's this for?
5. this thing	5. What's this thing?
/ðə/	
1. the best	1. The best is yet to come.
2. the last	2. Here's the last one.
3. the line	3. I draw the line here.
4. the game	4. The game just ended.
5. the one	5. He's the one!

Phrases	*Sentences*
/ði/	
1. these books	1. These books are heavy.
2. gave you these	2. Who gave you these?
3. all of these	3. We'll need all of these.
4. these days	4. These days, who knows?
5. put these	5. Put these away.
/ðe/	
1. they knew	1. They knew it all along.
2. they should	2. They should be here.
3. they say	3. That's what they say.
4. they tell me	4. They tell me you're free.
5. they think	5. Who do they think they are?
/ðaʊ/	
1. without you	1. I can't do it without you.
2. without me	2. Don't go without me.
3. without sugar	3. Without sugar, please.
4. come without	4. Don't come without calling.
5. without help	5. You can't do it without help.

/ð/ CONTEXTS

Distinctive features: linguadental (interdental), fricative-continuant, voiced
/ð/ ***vowel combinations:*** Initial position of an unstressed syllable

Deep Test

/ðɛ/ themselves /ðɚ/ another

Common Words

/ðɚ/	/ðɛ/
another	themselves
brother	
either	
father	
further	
gather	
mother	
neither	
other	
rather	
together	
weather	

Everyday Language

Phrases	*Sentences*
/ðɚ/	
1. another time	1. Do it another time.
2. either way	2. Either way is OK.
3. mother home	3. Is your mother home?
4. neither of us	4. Neither of us cares!
5. your brother	5. Where's your brother?
/ðɛ/	
1. do it themselves	1. They'll do it themselves.
2. know themselves	2. They know themselves best.
3. carry themselves	3. They carry themselves high.
4. kill themselves	4. They may kill themselves!
5. gave themselves	5. They gave themselves credit.

/ð/ CONTEXTS

Distinctive features: linguadental (interdental), fricative-continuant, voiced
/ð/ ***vowel combinations:*** Final position of a stressed syllable

Deep Test

/ɪð/ with

Common Words

/ɪð/

with

Everyday Language

Phrases	*Sentences*
/ɪð/	
1. she with	1. Who's she with?
2. with them	2. I came with them.
3. with this	3. Do it with this.
4. with the stripes	4. It's the one with the stripes.
5. with that	5. You won with that?

/s/ CONTEXTS

Distinctive features: linguaalveolar, fricative-continuant, voiceless
/s/ ***vowel combinations:*** Initial position of a stressed syllable

Deep Test

/si/ sea	/sɛ/ set	/sɔ/ saw	/su/ suit	/sʌ/ sun	/sɔɪ/ soil
/sɪ/ sit	/sæ/ sat	/so/ so	/sɝ/ sir	/saɪ/ side	/saʊ/ south
/se/ say					

Common Words

/sɛ/	/sɪ/	/sʌ/	/si/	/saɪ/	/sɝ/
accept	city	some	receive	beside	certain
cent	consider	something	scene	decide	certainly
center	sick	sometimes	season	outside	circle
century	silver	son	seat	side	serve
except	simple	subject	see	sight	service
herself	since	such	seek	sign	sir
himself	sing	suddenly	seem	silence	
itself	single	suffer	seen	size	
myself	sister	summer		society	
said	sit	sun			
second	six				
sell	system				
send					
sense					
sent					
settle					
seven					
several					
themselves					
yourself					

/se/	/sɔ/	/so/	/su/	/saʊ/	/sæ/	/sɔɪ/
safe	salt	so	soon	sound	sat	soil
sail	saw	sold	suit	south		
same	soft	soldier				
save	sort	soul				
say						

Everyday Language

Phrases	*Sentences*
/sɛ/	
1. need a cent	1. You don't need a cent.
2. who said	2. Who said so?
3. second best	3. You have to take second best.
4. sell anything	4. He can sell anything.
5. settle for less	5. We can't settle for less.

Phrases	*Sentences*
/sɪ/	
1. to the city	1. They moved to the city.
2. home sick	2. She's home sick today.
3. let's sing	3. Let's sing a duet.
4. my sister	4. My sister is here.
5. five times six	5. Five times six is _____.
/sʌ/	
1. sometimes it	1. Sometimes it isn't worth it.
2. one son	2. They have only one son.
3. it's such	3. It's such a fine line.
4. suddenly there	4. Suddenly there it was!
5. till summer	5. I can't wait till summer!
/si/	
1. the season	1. Tis the season to be jolly!
2. lose your seat	2. You may lose your seat.
3. I seem	3. I seem always to be late.
4. bad scene	4. It was a bad scene.
5. receive more	5. We should receive more.
/saɪ/	
1. can't decide	1. I can't decide what to wear.
2. waiting outside	2. She's waiting outside.
3. silence is golden	3. Silence is golden they say.
4. your size	4. It's just your size.
5. sit beside	5. Sit beside him and help.
/sɝ/	
1. form a circle	1. Let's form a circle
2. certainly look	2. You certainly look well.
3. certain of that	3. Are you certain of that?
4. service is poor	4. The service is poor.
5. help you sir	5. May I help you, sir?
/se/	
1. we'll sail	1. We'll sail there tomorrow.
2. save some	2. Better save some money.
3. couldn't say	3. I just couldn't say when.
4. be safe	4. It will be safe here.
5. it's the same	5. It's the same old thing!

Phrases	*Sentences*
/sɔ/	
1. more salt	1. Put in little more salt.
2. what sort	2. What sort of soup is that?
3. soft and warm	3. It's so soft and warm!
4. saw both	4. We saw both movies.
5. soft touch	5. You're a soft touch.
/so/	
1. so bad	1. It's not so bad.
2. sold out	2. They're all sold out.
3. my soul	3. Well, bless my soul!
4. soldier of fortune	4. He's a "soldier of fortune."
5. I sold	5. I sold my car.
/su/	
1. soon be	1. It'll soon be over.
2. new suit	2. That's a new suit.
3. back soon	3. Come back soon!
4. suit you	4. Fix it if it doesn't suit you.
5. as soon as	5. As soon as you can come in, do.
/saʊ/	
1. terrible sound	1. What a terrible sound!
2. from the south	2. She's from the south.
3. go south	3. Go south about three miles.
4. this sound	4. Try to say this sound.
5. sound it out	5. Maybe you can sound it out.
/sæ/	
1. sat through	1. We sat through the whole show.
2. sat by	2. She sat by me.
3. sat there	3. It just sat there!
4. sat forever	4. Seems like we sat forever!
5. sat still	5. They all sat still.
/sɔɪ/	
1. soil your dress	1. Did you soil your dress?
2. good soil	2. That's good soil.
3. potting soil	3. We need more potting soil.
4. this soil	4. This soil is too dry.
5. any soil	5. It'll grow in about any soil.

/s/ CONTEXTS

Distinctive features: linguaalveolar, fricative-continuant, voiceless
/s/ ***vowel combinations:*** Initial position of an unstressed syllable

Deep Test

/so/ also /sɚ/ answer /sə/ supply /saɪ/ exercise

Common Words

/sə/	/sɚ/	/so/	/saɪ/
listen	answer	also	exercise
passage	officer		
person			
possible			
society			
success			
supply			
suppose			

Everyday Language

Phrases	*Sentences*
/sə/	
1. nice person	1. She's a nice person.
2. supply store	2. Where's the art supply store?
3. I suppose	3. I suppose you want to keep it.
4. let success	4. Don't let success spoil it.
5. high society	5. You're in high society now.
/sɚ/	
1. answer me	1. Answer me now!
2. that officer	2. Ask that officer for help.
3. new officer	3. He's a new officer.
4. answer yet	4. Did they answer yet?
5. an answer today	5. We should get an answer today.
/so/	
1. also need	1. We'll also need a box.
2. go also	2. You may go also.
3. also like	3. I also like apples.
4. you also	4. Are you also a member?
5. also pay	5. Members also pay.

Phrases	*Sentences*
/saɪ/	
1. first exercise	1. Do the first exercise.
2. to exercise	2. I hate to exercise.
3. good exercise	3. That's good exercise.
4. more exercise	4. Finish one more exercise.
5. daily exercise	5. Daily exercise is important.

/s/ CONTEXTS

Distinctive features: linguaalveolar, fricative-continuant, voiceless
/s/ ***vowel combinations:*** Final position of a stressed syllable

Deep Test

/is/ peace	/ɛs/ yes	/os/ close	/ʌs/ us	/aʊs/ house
/ɪs/ kiss	/æs/ pass	/us/ produce	/aɪs/ ice	/ɔɪs/ voice
/es/ base	/ɔs/ loss			

Common Words

/ɛs/	/es/	/æs/	/ɪs/	/is/	/ɔs/	/aɪs/	/os/
dress	base	class	kiss	increase	across	ice	close
guess	case	glass	miss	peace	cross	nice	
less	face	grass	this	piece	loss	price	
press	place	pass					
question	race						
success	space						
unless							
yes							

/us/	/ʌs/	/aʊs/	/ɔɪs/
produce	us	house	voice

Everyday Language

Phrases	*Sentences*
/ɛs/	
1. dress up	1. Do we have to dress up?
2. the question	2. What's the question now?
3. that's less	3. That's less than I thought.
4. yes or no	4. Is the answer "yes" or "no"?
5. I guess	5. I guess I better go.
/es/	
1. touch base	1. Touch base first.
2. it's a case	2. It's a case of good timing.
3. our place	3. Come over to our place.
4. outer space	4. She's in outer space.
5. place for you	5. We have a place for you.
/æs/	
1. what class	1. What class are you in?
2. small glass	2. I'll have a small glass.
3. cut the grass	3. Time to cut the grass.
4. please pass	4. Please pass the mustard.
5. you'll pass	5. Do you think you'll pass?
/ɪs/	
1. miss is	1. A miss is as good as _____.
2. kiss me	2. Kiss me, you fool!
3. miss her	3. I really miss her.
4. this was	4. This was your last chance.
5. this is	5. This is really nice!
/is/	
1. increase in	1. They'll increase in price.
2. pray for peace	2. Let us all pray for peace.
3. a little piece	3. Give me just a little piece.
4. piece of cake	4. It's a piece of cake!
5. missing piece	5. What's the missing piece?
/ɔs/	
1. sit across	1. Sit across from me.
2. cross my heart	2. Cross my heart, it's true!
3. big loss	3. It's no big loss.
4. across the street	4. They just live across the street.
5. their loss	5. Our gain is their loss.

Phrases	*Sentences*
/aɪs/	
1. cold as ice	1. It's cold as ice!
2. more ice	2. May I have more ice?
3. it's nice	3. It's nice to see you.
4. good price	4. That's a good price.
5. the price	5. What's the price now?
/os/	
1. close race	1. It's a close race.
2. sit close	2. Sit close to me.
3. close call	3. That was a close call.
4. close friends	4. We're close friends.
5. feel close	5. I feel close to you.
/us/	
1. have to produce	1. You'll have to produce.
2. produce results	2. That will produce results.
3. we produce	3. We produce a good thing.
4. produce the evidence	4. Produce the evidence or else!
5. produce the facts	5. They'll produce the facts.
/ʌs/	
1. one of us	1. She's one of us.
2. all of us	2. All of us miss you.
3. give us	3. Give us a break!
4. happen to us	4. It could only happen to us!
5. gave us	5. He gave us a good excuse.
/aʊs/	
1. your house	1. Is this your house?
2. my house	2. My house is your house.
3. our house	3. Come over to our house.
4. building a house	4. They're building a house.
5. house on the corner	5. It's the house on the corner.
/ɔɪs/	
1. nice voice	1. She has a nice voice.
2. a full voice	2. It isn't a full voice.
3. your voice	3. Is that your voice?
4. my voice	4. My voice sounds different.
5. good voice	5. He's in good voice!

/s/ CONTEXTS

Distinctive features: linguaalveolar, fricative-continuant, voiceless
/s/ ***vowel combinations:*** Final position of an unstressed syllable

Deep Test

/ɪs/ discover /əs/ industry

Common Words

/ɪs/	/əs/
business	famous
discover	industry
notice	various
office	
practice	
promise	
purpose	
service	

Everyday Language

Phrases	*Sentences*
/ɪs/	
1. your business	1. What's your business?
2. gave you notice	2. They gave you notice yesterday.
3. my office	3. Come to my office.
4. promise you won't	4. Promise you won't tell.
5. notice it	5. Did you notice it?
/əs/	
1. famous now	1. You're famous now.
2. new industry	2. It's a new industry.
3. various sizes	3. They come in various sizes.
4. various times	4. It goes off at various times.
5. famous people	5. Famous people are nice.

/s/ CONTEXTS

Distinctive features: linguaalveolar, fricative-continuant, voiceless
/s/ ***blends:*** Initial position of a stressed syllable

Deep Test

/st/ star	/str/ street	/sm/ smile	/skw/ square	/sl/ sleep
/sp/ speech	/sk/ school	/spl/ explain	/sn/ snow	/sw/ sweet

Common Words

/st/	/sp/	/str/	/sk/	/sm/	/spl/
instead	especially	destroy	escape	small	explain
stand	expect	straight	school	smile	
star	experience	strange	skin	smoke	
start	space	stream	sky		
state	speak	street			
station	special	strength			
stay	speech				
step	spend				
stick	spirit				
still	spoke				
stock	spot				
stone					
stood					
stop					
store					
storm					
story					
study					
understood					

/skw/	/sn/	/sl/	/sw/
square	snow	sleep	sweet

Everyday Language

Phrases	*Sentences*
/st/	
1. start walking	1. Start walking, mister!
2. state your business	2. State your business and leave.
3. step right	3. Step right up, ma'm.
4. stick 'em	4. Stick 'em up!
5. the storm	5. The storm ruined it.

Phrases	*Sentences*
/sp/	
1. expect snow	1. They expect snow tonight.
2. short on space	2. We're a little short on space.
3. speak up	3. Well, speak up, man!
4. special program	4. This is a special program.
5. hits the spot	5. That really hits the spot!
/str/	
1. get it straight	1. Try to get it straight this time.
2. strange way	2. That's a strange way to do it, but OK!
3. destroy me	3. You just destroy me!
4. what street	4. What street do you live on?
5. be strong	5. Be strong; it'll soon be done.
/sk/	
1. no escape	1. There's no escape from it.
2. school starts	2. School starts again tomorrow.
3. my skin	3. My skin is so dry.
4. sky high	4. It went sky high!
5. skin him	5. I'd like to skin him!
/sm/	
1. a small favor	1. Do me a small favor?
2. smile awhile	2. "Smile awhile," they say.
3. don't smoke	3. Don't smoke here, please.
4. a small world	4. It's a small world.
5. smell smoke	5. I smell smoke!
/spl/	
1. explain it	1. I can't explain it.
2. explain yourself	2. You better explain yourself.
3. explain the game	3. Explain the game to us.
4. explain it all	4. I'll explain it all later.
5. can't explain	5. Some things you just can't explain.
/skw/	
1. a foot square	1. It's about a foot square.
2. isn't square	2. This really isn't square.
3. square dance	3. Do you square dance?
4. around the square	4. Drive around the square.
5. forty square miles	5. There are 40 square miles of water.

Phrases	*Sentences*
/sn/	
1. more snow	1. They predict more snow.
2. snow ski	2. Can you snow ski?
3. light snow	3. There's a light snow.
4. snow flurries	4. There are snow flurries now.
5. snow is melting.	5. The snow is melting fast.
/sl/	
1. get some sleep	1. Did you get some sleep?
2. sleep tight	2. Sleep tight now.
3. with sleep	3. You'll feel better with sleep.
4. should I sleep	4. Where should I sleep?
5. sleep late	5. She'll probably sleep late.
/sw/	
1. sweet music	1. That's sweet music.
2. awfully sweet	2. It's awfully sweet.
3. something sweet	3. I crave something sweet!
4. sweet thing	4. Hello, sweet thing!
5. you're sweet	5. You're sweet to do that for me.

/s/ CONTEXTS

Distinctive features: linguaalveolar, fricative-continuant, voiceless
/s/ ***blends:*** Initial position of an unstressed syllable

Deep Test

/st/ distance

Common Words

/st/

distance
history
master
sister
system

Everyday Language

Phrases	*Sentences*
/st/	
1. your sister	1. Is your sister coming?
2. the system	2. You have to learn the system.
3. master key	3. Who has the master key?
4. long distance	4. You have a long distance call.
5. history course	5. I hate my history course.

/s/ CONTEXTS

Distinctive features: linguaalveolar, fricative-continuant, voiceless
/s/ ***blends:*** Final position of a stressed syllable

Deep Test

/st/ best   /sk/ ask

Common Words

/st/	/sk/
best	ask
cost	
east	
fast	
first	
just	
last	
least	
lost	
most	
must	
past	
post	
rest	
suggest	
taste	
trust	
waste	
west	

Everyday Language

Phrases	*Sentences*
/st/	
1. my best suit	1. This is my best suit.
2. did it cost	2. How much did it cost?
3. got here first	3. I got here first.
4. last night	4. Last night I went to bed early.
5. that's the least	5. That's the least he could do.
/sk/	
1. ask him	1. Ask him tonight.
2. don't ask	2. Just don't ask!
3. hurt to ask	3. It won't hurt to ask.
4. is ask	4. All you can do is ask.
5. ask now	5. Why ask now?

/s/ CONTEXTS

Distinctive features: linguaalveolar, fricative-continuant, voiceless
/s/ ***blends:*** Final position of an unstressed syllable

Deep Test

/st/ almost

Common Words

/st/
almost
forest
interest

Everyday Language

Phrases	*Sentences*
/st/	
1. almost done	1. I'm almost done.
2. see the forest	2. You can't see the forest _____.
3. how much interest	3. How much interest is there?
4. little interest	4. There's little interest in it.
5. high interest	5. It pays a high interest.

/z/ CONTEXTS

Distinctive features: linguaalveolar, fricative-continuant, voiced
/z/ ***vowel combinations:*** Initial position of a stressed syllable

Deep Test

/zɪ/ position /zæ/ example /zʌ/ result /zaɪ/ desire

Common Words

/zɪ/	/zæ/	/zʌ/	/zaɪ/
position	example	result	desire

Everyday Language

Phrases	*Sentences*
/zɪ/	
1. position open	1. There's a position open.
2. that position	2. Hold that position!
3. position it	3. Position it near the window.
4. good position	4. You're in good position.
5. second position	5. You're in second position.
/zæ/	
1. good example	1. Set a good example.
2. poor example	2. This is a poor example.
3. example one	3. Example one is easy.
4. one more example	4. We need one more example.
5. an example	5. Give us an example.
/zʌ/	
1. poor result	1. We got a poor result.
2. will result	2. What will result from this?
3. result is	3. The result is progress.
4. predict the result	4. You can't predict the result.
5. one result	5. One result could be _____.
/zaɪ/	
1. no desire	1. I have no desire to go.
2. desire most	2. What do you desire most?
3. one desire	3. That's my one desire!
4. no real desire	4. They have no real desire to fight.
5. but one desire	5. If I had but one desire it would be _____.

/z/ CONTEXTS

Distinctive features: linguaalveolar, fricative-continuant, voiced
/z/ ***vowel combinations:*** Initial position of an unstressed syllable

Deep Test

/zɪ/ music /zə/ reason

Common Words

/zə/	/zɪ/
reason	music
season	
thousand	

Everyday Language

Phrases	*Sentences*
/zə/	
1. a good reason	1. That's not a good reason.
2. season it	2. Season it with sage.
3. been a thousand	3. There must have been a thousand.
4. reason is	4. The reason is this.
5. next season	5. Next season we'll do better.
/zɪ/	
1. hear music	1. I hear music!
2. that's music	2. That's music to my ears.
3. music was	3. The music was too loud.
4. her music	4. Her music is always good.
5. music major	5. She's a music major.

/z/ CONTEXTS

Distinctive features: linguaalveolar, fricative-continuant, voiced
/z/ ***vowel combinations:*** Final position of a stressed syllable

Deep Test

/iz/ these	/ez/ raise	/ɔz/ cause	/uz/ lose	/aɪz/ wise
/ɪz/ is	/æz/ as	/oz/ nose	/ʌz/ does	

Common Words

/uz/	/oz/	/aɪz/	/ɪz/	/ʌz/	/iz/
lose	clothes	rise	business	does	please
news	nose	size	his	husband	these
newspaper	rose	surprise	is	was	
refuse	suppose	wise			
use	those				
whose					

/æz/	/ɔz/	/ez/
as	cause	raise
has	because	

Everyday Language

Phrases	*Sentences*
/uz/	
1. lose the place	1. Don't lose the place.
2. no news	2. No news is good news.
3. good news	3. There's good news and bad news.
4. refuse me	4. You can't refuse me.
5. whose turn	5. Whose turn is it?
/oz/	
1. nice clothes	1. She wears nice clothes.
2. your nose	2. Don't turn up your nose!
3. rose is	3. A rose is a rose is . . .
4. I suppose	4. I suppose i can.
5. those people	5. Those people should help.
/aɪz/	
1. let it rise	1. Let it rise; then bake it.
2. what size	2. What size is this?
3. surprise them	3. Won't it surprise them?
4. wise to wait	4. You're wise to wait.
5. the size of it	5. That's about the size of it.
/ɪz/	
1. it's business	1. It's business as usual.
2. your business	2. None of your business!
3. his chance	3. He missed his chance.
4. is it	4. Well, this is it!
5. his turn	5. It's his turn to drive.

Phrases	*Sentences*
/ʌz/	
1. does the train	1. Does the train stop here?
2. your husband	2. Your husband called.
3. what was	3. What was that all about?
4. who was	4. Who was that?
5. does help?	5. Money does help!
/iz/	
1. these people	1. Who are these people?
2. more coffee please	2. I'd like more coffee please.
3. these are	3. These are very helpful.
4. please me	4. That would please me.
5. please her	5. That didn't please her.
/æz/	
1. bright as day	1. It's as bright as day.
2. who has	2. Who has the hammer?
3. has a way	3. She has a way about her.
4. may as well	4. We may as well go.
5. has it stopped	5. Has it stopped raining?
/ɔz/	
1. a good cause	1. It's for a good cause.
2. may cause	2. It may cause a fuss.
3. because it's for	3. Because it's for you, I'll do it.
4. came because	4. We came because we're needed.
5. no cause	5. There's no cause for alarm.
/ez/	
1. they'll raise	1. They'll raise the dickens!
2. get a raise	2. Did you get a raise?
3. raise it	3. Raise it a bit more.
4. raise the window	4. Raise the window before you leave.
5. raise your hand	5. Raise your hand before you speak.

/z/ CONTEXTS

Distinctive features: linguaalveolar, fricative-continuant, voiced
/z/ ***vowel combinations:*** Final position of an unstressed syllable

Deep Test

/ez/ always /aɪz/ realize

Common Words

/aɪz/	/ez/
exercise	always
realize	

Everyday Language

Phrases	*Sentences*
/aɪz/	
1. didn't realize	1. I didn't realize how fast!
2. you realize	2. Do you realize what you're doing?
3. my exercise	3. My exercise went quickly.
4. graduation exercise	4. The graduation exercise is today.
5. must exercise	5. You must exercise your rights.
/ez/	
1. always ask	1. Always ask permission first.
2. always late	2. You're always late!
3. always me	3. Why is it always me?
4. love you always	4. I'll love you always!
5. always tell	5. You can't always tell.

/ʃ/ CONTEXTS

Distinctive features: linguapalatal, fricative-continuant, voiceless
/ʃ/ ***vowel combinations:*** Initial position of a stressed syllable

Deep Test

/ʃi/ she	/ʃɛ/ share	/ʃa/ shop	/ʃɔ/ show	/ʃu/ shoe
/ʃɪ/ ship	/ʃæ/ shall	/ʃɔ/ short	/ʃʊ/ should	/ʃaʊ/ shout
/ʃe/ shape				

Common Words

/ʃo/	/ʃi/	/ʃe/	/ʃa/	/ʃɪ/	/ʃɛ/	/ʃæ/	/ʃɔ/
shore	machine	shade	shop	ship	share	shall	short
shoulder	she	shape	shot				
show							

/ʃʊ/	/ʃu/	/ʃaʊ/
should	shoe	shout

Everyday Language

Phrases	*Sentences*
/ʃo/	
1. to the shore	1. We're going to the shore.
2. swim to shore	2. Swim to shore now.
3. your shoulder	3. Move your shoulder.
4. show us	4. Show us how you do it.
5. big showoff	5. He's a big showoff.
/ʃi/	
1. new machine	1. They got a new machine.
2. she can't	2. She can't be here.
3. machine shop	3. The machine shop has it.
4. better get	4. She'd better get busy!
5. she going	5. Is she going or not?
/ʃe/	
1. in the shade	1. It's about 90° in the shade.
2. under the shade	2. Let's sit under the shade.
3. what shape	3. What shape is it in?
4. bad shape	4. You're in bad shape.
5. a shade darker	5. Make it a shade darker.
/ʃa/	
1. shop awhile	1. Let's shop awhile.
2. a shot	2. Was that a shot?
3. heard the shot	3. He heard the shot too.
4. shop closed	4. The shop is closed today.
5. open the shop	5. They open the shop at nine.
/ʃɪ/	
1. ship sails	1. The ship sails at noon.
2. ship it	2. We'll ship it collect.
3. ship out	3. Shape up or ship out!
4. my ship	4. When will my ship come in?
5. ship everything	5. They ship everything anywhere.
/ʃɛ/	
1. learn to share	1. You must learn to share.
2. their share	2. They got their share.
3. fair share	3. Is that a fair share?
4. share my seat	4. Share my seat, please?
5. share a sandwich	5. Will you share a sandwich?

Phrases	*Sentences*
/ʃæ/	
1. what shall	1. What shall we do?
2. shall I	2. Shall I call you?
3. shall not	3. I shall not forget.
4. you shall	4. You shall not tell.
5. we shall	5. We shall be there.
/ʃɔ/	
1. too short	1. He's too short.
2. the short one	2. Give me the short one.
3. short drink	3. I'll have a short drink.
4. short stop	4. Who's playing short stop?
5. little short	5. We're a little short this month.
/ʃU/	
1. I should	1. I should be going.
2. pass the sugar	2. Pass the sugar, please.
3. sugar is	3. Sugar is sweet and _____.
4. should this	4. Should this be here?
5. should say	5. Well, I should say so!
/ʃu/	
1. other shoe	1. Drop the other shoe!
2. black shoe	2. Where's my black shoe?
3. shoe fits	3. If the shoe fits _____.
4. a shoe store	4. He runs a shoe store.
5. this shoe	5. This shoe is too tight.
/ʃaU/	
1. have to shout	1. You don't have to shout!
2. shout out	2. Shout out your name.
3. loud shout	3. A loud shout will do it.
4. you shout	4. We heard you shout.
5. a shout	5. Was that a shout?

/ʃ/ CONTEXTS

Distinctive features: linguapalatal, fricative-continuant, voiceless
/ʃ/ ***vowel combinations:*** Initial position of an unstressed syllable

Deep Test

/ʃə/ action /ʃu/ issue

Common Words

/ʃə/	/ʃu/
action	issue
attention	
condition	
direction	
especially	
nation	
national	
ocean	
position	
special	
station	

Everyday Language

Phrases	*Sentences*
/ʃə/	
1. take action	1. They take action quickly!
2. attention everyone	2. Attention, everyone, attention!
3. ocean is	3. The ocean is awesome.
4. at the station	4. We'll meet at the station.
5. lose direction	5. Did you lose direction?
/ʃu/	
1. big issue	1. What's the big issue?
2. the issue	2. The issue is money.
3. first issue	3. Is this the first issue?
4. an issue	4. Don't make an issue of it.
5. issue stamps	5. Where do they issue stamps?

/ʃ/ CONTEXTS

Distinctive features: linguapalatal, fricative-continuant, voiceless
/ʃ/ ***vowel combinations:*** Final position of a stressed syllable

Deep Test

/ɪʃ/ fish　　/ɛʃ/ fresh　　/ɔʃ/ wash　　/ʌʃ/ rush

Common Words

/ɪʃ/	/ɛʃ/	/ʌʃ/	/ɔʃ/
fish	fresh	rush	wash
wish			

Everyday Language

Phrases	*Sentences*
/ɪʃ/	
1. big fish	1. Who caught the big fish?
2. fish around	2. Just fish around a bit.
3. wish you	3. I wish you luck!
4. I wish	4. I wish I'd gone.
5. my wish	5. That's my wish, too.
/ɛʃ/	
1. fresh bread	1. I smell fresh bread.
2. fresh air	2. Fresh air feels good.
3. feel fresh	3. I feel fresh and rested.
4. get fresh	4. Don't get fresh!
5. fresh start	5. Get a fresh start.
/ʌʃ/	
1. don't rush	1. Don't rush through it.
2. rush is on	2. Well, the rush is on!
3. can't rush	3. You can't rush it.
4. in the rush	4. We're caught in the rush.
5. rush it	5. Rush it over here.
/ɔʃ/	
1. wash your face	1. Wash your face and hands.
2. car wash	2. Where's the car wash?
3. do the wash	3. I need to do the wash.
4. wash up	4. Wash up before dinner.
5. the wash room	5. Here's the wash room.

/ʃ/ CONTEXTS

Distinctive features: linguapalatal, fricative-continuant, voiceless
/ʃ/ vowel combinations: Final position of an unstressed syllable

Deep Test

/ɪʃ/ finish

Common Words

/ɪʃ/
finish

Everyday Language

Phrases

/ɪʃ/

1. at the finish
2. you finish
3. can't finish
4. finish tonight
5. tough finish

Sentences

1. They're at the finish!
2. Did you finish?
3. I can't finish.
4. We'll finish tonight.
5. It's a tough finish.

/ʒ/ CONTEXTS

Distinctive features: linguapalatal, fricative-continuant, voiced
/ʒ/ vowel combinations: Initial position of an unstressed syllable

Deep Test

/ʒɚ/ measure /ʒə/ usually

Common Words

/ʒɚ/	/ʒə/
measure	usually
pleasure	

Everyday Language

Phrases	*Sentences*
/ʒɚ/	
1. measure it	1. We'd better measure it.
2. measure up	2. It doesn't measure up.
3. your pleasure	3. What's your pleasure?
4. pleasure trip	4. This is a pleasure trip.
5. full measure	5. They give you full measure.
/ʒə/	
1. usually eat	1. We usually eat here.
2. usually quiet	2. It's usually quiet.
3. usually shy	3. I'm not usually shy.
4. usually helps	4. Who usually helps you?
5. usually on	5. You're usually on time.

/h/ CONTEXTS

Distinctive features: glottal, fricative-continuant, voiceless
/h/ ***vowel combinations:*** Initial position of a stressed syllable

Deep Test

/hi/ he	/hæ/ had	/hɔ/ hall	/hɝ/ her	/haɪ/ high
/hɪ/ him	/hɑ/ hot	/ho/ hole	/hʌ/ hundred	/haʊ/ how
/hɛ/ head				

Common Words

/hæ/	/hɛ/	/hɪ/	/ho/	/hɝ/	/haɪ/	/hɑ/	/hi/
had	hair	hear	hold	heard	behind	hard	he
half	head	here	hole	her	height	heart	heat
hand	health	hill	home	hurry	high	hot	
hang	heaven	him	hope	hurt			
happen	heavy	his					
happy	held	history					
has	help						
hat							

/hʌ/	/haʊ/	/hɔ/
hundred	house	hall
husband	how	

Everyday Language

Phrases	*Sentences*
/hæ/	
1. had it	1. I've had it!
2. take half	2. You take half.
3. have to hand	3. You have to hand it to him.
4. happen now	4. Anything can happen now.
5. really happy	5. Are you really happy?
/hɛ/	
1. your hair	1. Your hair is a mess!
2. get to heaven	2. You'll never get to heaven that way!
3. heavy for	3. This is heavy for me.
4. good health	4. Good health to you!
5. your head	5. Use your head now.
/hɪ/	
1. hear the news	1. Did you hear the news?
2. here it comes	2. Get ready, here it comes!
3. history repeats	3. History repeats itself.
4. give him	4. Just give him time.
5. up hill	5. It's all up hill now.
/ho/	
1. hold it	1. Hold it there!
2. in the hole	2. I'm two dollars in the hole.
3. to get home	3. It's good to get home.
4. hope you win	4. Hope you win next time.
5. hold on	5. Hold on, here we go!
/hɝ/	
1. we heard	1. We heard you were here.
2. give her	2. Give her credit for trying.
3. hurry now	3. Hurry now, don't be late.
4. won't hurt	4. It won't hurt to try.
5. heard the news	5. Have you heard the news?
/haɪ/	
1. behind time	1. You're behind time.
2. the right height	2. That's about the right height.
3. too high	3. Prices are too high.
4. from behind	4. They came from behind to win.
5. a high time	5. We had a high time!

Phrases

/hɑ/

1. hard to
2. have a heart
3. hot dog
4. heart to heart
5. hard times

/hi/

1. won't he
2. beat the heat
3. he won't
4. more heat
5. he came

/hʌ/

1. a hundred dollars
2. your husband
3. on a hundred
4. my husband
5. a hundred to

/haʊ/

1. my house
2. how do you
3. how are you
4. show me how
5. next house

/hɔ/

1. of the hall
2. which hall
3. sweep the hall
4. at the hall
5. in the hall

Sentences

/hɑ/

1. It's hard to tell.
2. Have a heart, lend me a dollar!
3. Here's a hot dog.
4. We should have a heart to heart talk.
5. Hard times may never come.

/hi/

1. Won't he be surprised?
2. How can you beat the heat?
3. He won't tell us.
4. More heat would help.
5. He came, he saw, he . . .

/hʌ/

1. Bet you a hundred dollars!
2. Your husband can come, too.
3. Plan on a hundred at least.
4. Did my husband call?
5. It's a hundred-to-one chance.

/haʊ/

1. Come to my house.
2. How do you manage?
3. How are you doing?
4. Show me how you do it, OK?
5. It's the next house.

/hɔ/

1. Go to the end of the hall.
2. Which hall do you live in?
3. We need to sweep the hall.
4. Is the dance at the hall?
5. We'll meet in the hall.

/h/ CONTEXTS

Distinctive features: glottal, fricative-continuant, voiceless
/h/ ***vowel combinations:*** Initial position of an unstressed syllable

Deep Test

/hɪ/ himself   /hɚ/ herself   /haʊ/ however

Common Words

/hɪ/	/hɚ/	/haʊ/
himself	herself	however

Everyday Language

Phrases	*Sentences*
/hɪ/	
1. go himself	1. He'll have to go himself.
2. has himself	2. He has himself to blame.
3. knows himself	3. He knows himself.
4. by himself	4. He came by himself.
5. hates himself	5. He hates himself for it.
/hɚ/	
1. go herself	1. She'll have to go herself.
2. herself to blame	2. She has herself to blame.
3. knows herself	3. She knows herself.
4. by herself	4. She came by herself.
5. hates herself	5. She hates herself for it.
/haʊ/	
1. however you may	1. However, you may be mistaken.
2. the same however	2. We all want the same, however.
3. however it comes	3. However it comes out is alright.
4. over however	4. We knew it was over, however.
5. however did	5. However did you guess?

/hw/ CONTEXTS

Distinctive features: glottal-bilabial, fricative, voiceless to half-voiced
/hw/ ***vowel combinations:*** Initial position of a stressed syllable

Deep Test

/hwɪ/ which /hwɛ/ when /hwɑ/ what /hwaɪ/ why

Common Words

/hwɛ/	/hwaɪ/	/hwɪ/	/hwɑ/
when	while	which	what
where	white		
whether	why		

Everyday Language

Phrases	*Sentences*
/hwɛ/	
1. when did you	1. When did you get here?
2. where are you	2. Where are you staying?
3. whether we like it	3. Whether we like it or not, I guess.
4. say when	4. He didn't say when.
5. know where	5. He didn't know where either.
/hwaɪ/	
1. while you	1. While you were out, he called.
2. white walls	2. I prefer white walls.
3. why don't	3. Why don't you ever call?
4. know why	4. I really don't know why.
5. while I listen	5. You talk while I listen.
/hwɪ/	
1. which way	1. Which way did he go?
2. which dress	2. Which dress did you wear?
3. which book	3. Which book did you read?
4. which one	4. She didn't say which one.
5. which is biggest	5. Tell me which is biggest.

Phrases

/hwɑ/

1. what time
2. what to say
3. what was
4. what he heard
5. what day

Sentences

1. What time is it?
2. I don't know what to say.
3. What was that noise?
4. Ask him what he heard.
5. What day is it due?

/hw/ CONTEXTS

Distinctive features: glottal-bilabial, fricative, voiceless to half-voiced
/hw/ ***vowel combinations:*** Initial position of an unstressed syllable

Deep Test

/hwə/ whatever

Common Words

/hwə/
whatever

Everyday Language

Phrases

/hwə/

1. whatever happens
2. do whatever
3. whatever we do
4. whatever we owe
5. whatever was that

Sentences

1. Whatever happens, I'll call.
2. Do whatever you wish.
3. Whatever we do, it's alright.
4. Whatever we owe, I'll pay.
5. Whatever was that sound?

/w/ CONTEXTS

Distinctive features: bilabial, nonfricative-glide, voiced (semivowel)
/w/ ***vowel combinations:*** Initial position of a stressed syllable

Deep Test

/wi/ we	/we/ way	/wɑ/ water	/wʊ/ wood	/wʌ/ was
/wɪ/ will	/wɛ/ wear	/wɔ/ wall	/wɝ/ were	/waɪ/ wide

Common Words

/wɪ/	/we/	/wɛ/	/wɝ/	/wɑ/	/wɔ/	/waɪ/
will	away	wear	were	want	walk	wide
win	wait	weather	word	wash	wall	wife
wind	waste	well	work	watch	war	wild
window	wave	went	world	water	warm	wise

/wʌ/	/wʊ/	/wi/
was	woman	we
wonder	wood	week
wonderful	would	

Everyday Language

Phrases	*Sentences*
/wɪ/	
1. I will	1. I will if you will.
2. winter is	2. Winter is a great time of year.
3. I wish	3. I wish he'd call.
4. women are	4. Women are really _____.
5. out the window	5. Look out the window.
/we/	
1. go away	1. Oh, go away, please!
2. wait for me	2. Wait for me downstairs.
3. waste not	3. Waste not, want not!
4. lose weight	4. I need to lose weight.
5. which way	5. Which way did they go?

Phrases	*Sentences*
/wɛ/	
1. weather has been	1. The weather has been great.
2. well I can't	2. Well, I can't say for sure.
3. go west	3. Go west, young man!
4. went west	4. He went west yesterday.
5. we wear	5. What should we wear?
/wɝ/	
1. have a word	1. May I have a word with you?
2. work out	2. It'll work out OK.
3. big world	3. It's a big world.
4. worth it	4. I hope it's worth it.
5. were you	5. Where were you yesterday?
/wɑ/	
1. wash up	1. Wash up for lunch.
2. watch your step	2. Watch your step going out.
3. water all	3. Water all the plants.
4. want to	4. Want to help me?
5. my watch	5. My watch has stopped.
/wɔ/	
1. walk right	1. Walk right on by.
2. to the wall	2. My back's to the wall.
3. a war on	3. Looks like there's a war on.
4. plenty warm	4. I'm plenty warm now.
5. walk will	5. A walk will do you good.
/waɪ/	
1. my wife	1. Is my wife here?
2. wild place	2. This is a wild place!
3. be wise	3. Be wise, study hard.
4. wide place	4. There's a wide place ahead
5. too wild	5. Don't get too wild.
/wʌ/	
1. no wonder	1. It's no wonder to me.
2. it's wonderful	2. It's wonderful to be here.
3. was right	3. He was right about that.
4. just wonder	4. Don't you just wonder sometimes.
5. it was	5. It was no surprise.

Phrases / *Sentences*

/wʊ/

Phrases	Sentences
1. good woman	1. She's a good woman.
2. would you	2. Would you be able to help?
3. I would	3. I would if I could.
4. lovely wood	4. That's lovely wood.
5. needs a woman	5. It needs a woman to fix it.

/wi/

Phrases	Sentences
1. we can't	1. We can't be sure.
2. a week is	2. A week is a long time.
3. week after next	3. Week after next will be OK.
4. we ask	4. Whom will we ask?
5. in a week	5. There are only seven days in a week!

/w/ CONTEXTS

Distinctive features: bilabial, nonfricative-glide, voiced (semivowel)
/w/ ***vowel combinations:*** Initial position of an unstressed syllable

Deep Test

/wɪ/ within /we/ always /wɚ/ forward

Common Words

/wɪ/	/we/	/wɚ/
within	always	forward
without		

Everyday Language

/wɪ/

Phrases	*Sentences*
1. not within	1. It's not within his power.
2. go without you	2. We can't go without you.
3. come from within	3. It has to come from within.
4. fun without you	4. There's no fun without you.
5. within possibility	5. It's within possibility

Phrases	*Sentences*
/we/	
1. always happens	1. It always happens that way.
2. always stop	2. You can always stop.
3. always knew it	3. I always knew it would happen.
4. always is	4. Always is a long time.
5. always be	5. Always be on time.
/wɚ/	
1. too forward	1. That's being too forward.
2. sometimes forward	2. It's sometimes forward, sometimes back.
3. forward motion	3. A little forward motion helps.
4. move it forward	4. Move it forward about a foot.
5. forward thinking	5. That's forward thinking, it seems.

/l/ CONTEXTS

Distinctive features: linguaalveolar, latenal-nonfricative-continuant, voiced
/l/ ***vowel combinations:*** Initial position of a stressed syllable

Deep Test

/li/ leave	/lɛ/ let	/lɔ/ law	/lʊ/ look	/lɝ/ learn	/laɪ/ lie
/lɪ/ lip	/læ/ laugh	/lo/ low	/lu/ lose	/lʌ/ love	/laʊ/ allow
/le/ lay	/lɑ/ lot				

Common Words

/lɛ/	/le/	/lɔ/	/li/	/lɪ/	/laɪ/	/lo/	/læ/
led	lay	along	believe	lift	lie	alone	laugh
left	labor	belong	lead	lip	life	below	land
leg	lady	law	leader	listen	light	low	last
length	laid	long	least	little	like	lower	
less	lake	loss	leave	live	line		
let	late	lost					
letter							
unless							

/lɑ/	/lʊ/	/lu/	/lɝ/	/lʌ/	/laʊ/
large	look	lose	learn	love	allow
lot					

Everyday Language

Phrases	*Sentences*
/lɛ/	
1. left hand	1. Use your left hand.
2. take less	2. You wouldn't take less?
3. her letter	3. Her letter came today.
4. you tell	4. I won't unless you tell me.
5. led us	5. He's led us many times.
/le/	
1. lay it down	1. You better lay it down.
2. very late	2. It's getting very late.
3. to the lake	3. Let's go to the lake.
4. hard labor	4. That's hard labor.
5. laid plans	5. We've laid plans for it.
/lɔ/	
1. along the beach	1. Let's walk along the beach.
2. new law	2. There's a new law about that.
3. a long day	3. It's been a long day!
4. lost the key	4. We lost the key.
5. your loss	5. Your loss is our gain.
/li/	
1. I believe	1. I believe it could happen.
2. you lead	2. You lead, I'll follow.
3. who was leader	3. Who was leader last time?
4. the least	4. That's the least you could do.
5. leave me	5. Don't leave me here alone.
/lɪ/	
1. lift it	1. Lift it a little higher.
2. a fat lip	2. Want a fat lip?
3. listen to	3. Listen to her for once.
4. little longer	4. Just a little longer now.
5. we live	5. We live very well.
/laɪ/	
1. don't lie	1. Don't lie to me!
2. lie down	2. You'd better lie down.
3. that's life	3. Well, that's life!
4. the light	4. The light went off.
5. next line	5. Read the next line.

Phrases	*Sentences*
/lo/	
1. not alone	1. You're not alone, you know.
2. below zero	2. It's below zero now.
3. hold it lower	3. Hold it lower for me.
4. price is low	4. The price is low now.
5. below average	5. You're a little below average.
/læ/	
1. someone laugh	1. Did someone laugh?
2. make me laugh	2. Don't make me laugh!
3. see land	3. I see land over there.
4. the last one	4. This is the last one.
5. last year	5. My last year was best.
/lɑ/	
1. large order	1. That's a large order.
2. a lot	2. I like you a lot.
3. lot of people	3. A lot of people are going.
4. large size	4. He takes a large size.
5. large one	5. Buy the large one.
/lʊ/	
1. look up	1. Look up at the ceiling.
2. look down	2. Now look down.
3. look to the left	3. Look to the left, please.
4. look to the right	4. Look to the right, please
5. look straight	5. Now look straight ahead.
/lɝ/	
1. ever learn	1. Won't she ever learn?
2. live and learn	2. We live and learn.
3. learn something	3. I always learn something.
4. learn that	4. Where did you learn that?
5. slow to learn	5. He's slow to learn.
/lʌ/	
1. love makes	1. Love makes us happy.
2. just love	2. I just love children!
3. love it	3. Don't you just love it?
4. we'd love	4. We'd love to have you.
5. I'd love	5. I'd love to be there.

Phrases	*Sentences*
/laʊ/	
1. allow pets	1. They don't allow pets.
2. I allow	2. I allow as how they do.
3. allow it	3. She won't allow it.
4. they'll allow	4. They'll allow two chances.
5. allow you	5. I just can't allow you to go.
/lu/	
1. lose it	1. Did you lose it?
2. win or lose	2. You either win or lose.
3. if you lose	3. Don't cry if you lose!
4. we lose	4. If we lose, I'll die!
5. lose again	5. I'm sure they'll lose again.

/l/ CONTEXTS

Distinctive features: linguaalveolar, lateral-nonfricative-continuant, voiced
/l/ ***vowel combinations:*** Initial position of an unstressed syllable

Deep Test

/lɪ/ early /lə/ silence /laɪ/ realize /lo/ follow /lɚ/ color

Common Words

/lɪ/	/lo/	/lə/	/lɚ/	/laɪ/
certainly	fellow	island	color	realize
college	follow	problem	dollar	
daily	following	silence		
early	yellow			
family				
knowledge				
nearly				
only				
public				
quickly				
suddenly				
valley				
village				

Everyday Language

Phrases	*Sentences*
/lɪ/	
1. daily exercise	1. My daily exercise helps.
2. early to bed	2. Early to bed and early to rise . . .
3. only knows	3. Heaven only knows!
4. come quickly	4. Come quickly now!
5. suddenly felt	5. I suddenly felt faint.
/lo/	
1. nice fellow	1. He's a nice fellow.
2. follow me	2. Follow me closely.
3. following me	3. Are you following me?
4. yellow pages	4. Look in the yellow pages.
5. that fellow	5. Who's that fellow over there?
/lə/	
1. your problem	1. Your problem is money!
2. silence was	2. The silence was deafening!
3. an island	3. No man is an island.
4. the problem	4. The problem can be solved.
5. have silence	5. Could we have silence?
/lɚ/	
1. costs a dollar	1. It costs a dollar.
2. a dollar	2. Bet you a dollar I won!
3. color TV	3. Do you have a color TV?
4. favorite color	4. My favorite color is ______.
5. terrible color	5. That's a terrible color!
/laɪ/	
1. I realize	1. I realize what happened.
2. do you realize	2. Do you realize what day it is?
3. can realize	3. You can realize your dream.
4. realize success	4. Now you can realize success.
5. realize what	5. Do you realize what you're saying?

/l/ CONTEXTS

Distinctive features: linguaalveolar, lateral-nonfricative-continuant, voiced
/l/ ***vowel combinations:*** Final position of a stressed syllable

Deep Test

/il/ feel	/ɛl/ tell	/ol/ coal	/ul/ cool	/aɪl/ while
/ɪl/ ill	/æl/ shall	/ʊl/ full	/ɝl/ girl	/ɔɪl/ oil
/el/ fail	/ɔl/ all			

Common Words

/ɪl/	/ɔl/	/ol/	/ɛl/	/ul/	/el/	/æl/
bill	all	coal	fell	cool	fail	shall
children	almost	control	sell	fool	railroad	value
fill	also	hole	tell	rule	sail	
hill	always	roll	well	school		
ill	call	shoulder				
kill	fall	soldier				
million	hall	soul				
silver	small					
still	tall					
till	wall					
will						

/il/	/aɪl/	/ʊl/	/ɔɪl/	/ɝl/
deal	smile	full	oil	girl
feel	while	pull	soil	

Everyday Language

Phrases	*Sentences*
/ɪl/	
1. the bill	1. Send me the bill.
2. fill it	2. Fill it up, please.
3. so still	3. It's so still!
4. will there	4. Will there be anyone there?
5. little ill	5. You look a little ill.

Phrases	*Sentences*
/ɔl/	
1. all out	1. We're all out.
2. call first	2. You better call first.
3. don't fall	3. Watch and don't fall.
4. small chance	4. There's a small chance.
5. how tall	5. How tall are you?
/ol/	
1. burns coal	1. It burns coal.
2. like a roll	2. Would you like a roll?
3. hole in it	3. Now there's a hole in it.
4. my soul	4. Bless my soul!
5. move the control	5. Move the control over.
/ɛl/	
1. feel well	1. Don't you feel well?
2. fell out	2. It just fell out.
3. sell anything	3. You can sell anything.
4. tell me	4. Tell me how it happened.
5. you sell	5. Did you sell your car?
/ul/	
1. for school	1. Time for school now.
2. cool off	2. Cool off awhile here.
3. no rule	3. There's no rule about that.
4. cool spot	4. Here's a cool spot.
5. rule that out	5. Don't rule that out yet.
/el/	
1. won't fail	1. You won't fail this time.
2. like to sail	2. Do you like to sail?
3. we sail	3. We sail a great deal.
4. no railroad	4. There's no railroad there.
5. without fail	5. He comes without fail.
/æl/	
1. good value	1. Here's a good value.
2. you value	2. Do you value your life?
3. what shall	3. What shall we call it?
4. shall we	4. Shall we stop here?
5. we shall	5. We shall overcome!

Phrases	*Sentences*
/il/	
1. a raw deal	1. You got a raw deal.
2. feel bad	2. Don't you feel bad?
3. don't feel	3. I don't feel anything.
4. deal me in	4. Well deal me in, too!
5. closed the deal	5. They closed the deal today.
/ʊl/	
1. full house	1. It's a full house.
2. pull it	2. Pull it a little tighter.
3. lot of pull	3. He has a lot of pull here.
4. full talk	4. There's a full tank.
5. need a pull	5. We'll need a pull to get started.
/aɪl/	
1. to smile	1. Try to smile a little.
2. while we drive	2. We'll talk while we drive.
3. lovely smile	3. You have a lovely smile.
4. while I	4. They came while I was gone.
5. smile when	5. Smile when you say that!
/ɔɪl/	
1. quart of oil	1. Put in a quart of oil.
2. soil your shirt	2. You'll soil your shirt.
3. has the oil	3. Who has the oil?
4. rich in oil	4. He got rich in oil.
5. test the soil	5. Did they test the soil first?
/ɝl/	
1. girl friend	1. She's my girl friend.
2. baby girl	2. They had a baby girl.
3. for a girl	3. That's for a girl.
4. my girl	4. My girl can't go.
5. good girl	5. She's a good girl.

/l/ CONTEXTS

Distinctive features: linguaalveolar, lateral-nonfricative-continuant, voiced
/l/ ***vowel combinations:*** Final position of an unstressed syllable

Deep Test

/ɔl/ already /əl/ wonderful

Common Words

/əl/	/ɔl/
beautiful	already
general	although
material	
natural	
real	
really	
special	
usually	
wonderful	

Everyday Language

Phrases	*Sentences*
/əl/	
1. general rule	1. The general rule is in effect.
2. your own material	2. You need your own material.
3. really cold	3. It's really cold.
4. wonderful music	4. What wonderful music!
5. special teacher	5. She's a special teacher.
/ɔl/	
1. already gone	1. They're already gone.
2. although I don't	2. I would, although I don't want to.
3. already too many	3. There are already too many.
4. although he's finished	4. He'll come although he's finished.
5. already sold	5. That's already sold.

/l/ CONTEXTS

Distinctive features: linguaalveolar, lateral-nonfricative-continuant, voiced
/l/ ***blends:*** Final position of a stressed syllable

Deep Test

/ld/ cold	/lt/ built	/lk/ milk	/lvz/ themselves	/lθ/ health
/lf/ herself	/lp/ help	/lv/ twelve	/ls/ else	

Common Words

/ld/	/lf/	/lt/	/lp/	/lv/	/lvz/	/ls/
build	herself	built	help	twelve	themselves	else
child	himself	felt				
cold	itself	result				
field	myself	salt				
gold	yourself					
held						
hold						
old						
sold						
told						
wild						
world						

/lθ/	/lk/
health	milk

Everyday Language

Phrases	*Sentences*
/ld/	
1. cold out	1. It's really cold out!
2. good as gold	2. It's as good as gold.
3. an old story	3. That's an old story.
4. wild party	4. That was a wild party!
5. in the world	5. Where in the world are you?
/lf/	
1. do it yourself	1. Do it yourself today.
2. asked myself	2. I asked myself "why?"
3. all for himself	3. He kept it all for himself.
4. for herself	4. She's looking out for herself.
5. corrects itself	5. It corrects itself each day.
/lt/	
1. well-built house	1. It's a well-built house.
2. hasn't felt well	2. She hasn't felt well.
3. could result	3. That could result in disaster!
4. salt and pepper	4. Pass the salt and pepper.
5. a little salt	5. It needs a little salt.

Phrases	*Sentences*
/lp/	
1. help is	1. Help is on its way.
2. yell for help	2. Quick, yell for help!
3. no help needed	3. The sign says "No Help Needed."
4. help her out	4. Help her out if you can.
5. think would help	5. What do you think would help?
/lv/	
1. struck twelve	1. The clock struck twelve.
2. more than twelve	2. There are more than twelve here.
3. twelve times twelve	3. Twelve times twelve is _____.
4. twelve people	4. They picked twelve people.
5. only twelve	5. He's only twelve.
/lvz/	
1. helped themselves	1. They just helped themselves.
2. call themselves	2. They call themselves singers.
3. control themselves	3. They should control themselves.
4. blame themselves	4. They can only blame themselves.
5. they have themselves	5. They have themselves to thank.
/ls/	
1. what else	1. What else is there?
2. where else	2. Where else can we go?
3. so what else	3. So what else is new!
4. no one else	4. No one else wants it.
5. or else	5. Be there or else!
/lθ/	
1. watch your health	1. You must watch your health.
2. health foods	2. Health foods taste funny.
3. his health	3. His health is poor.
4. public health	4. She's in public health.
5. health club	5. Let's join a health club.
/lk/	
1. milk and eggs	1. Get some milk and eggs.
2. like milk	2. I don't like milk.
3. skim milk	3. She always drinks skim milk.
4. is milk	4. Is milk fattening?
5. goat's milk	5. Have you tasted goat's milk?

/r/ CONTEXTS

Distinctive features: linguaalveolar, retroflex-glide, voiced (semivowel)
/r/ ***vowel combinations:*** Initial position of a stressed syllable

Deep Test

/ri/ real	/re/ race	/ræ/ ran	/ro/ road	/ru/ room	/raɪ/ ride
/rɪ/ rich	/rɛ/ red	/rɑ/ rock	/rɔ/ wrong	/rʌ/ run	/raʊ/ round

Common Words

/rɛ/	/ri/	/re/	/raɪ/	/rɪ/	/ro/	/ru/
already	read	race	arrive	rich	road	rule
direct	real	railroad	ride	ring	rose	roof
direction	realize	rain	right	river	roll	
ready	really	raise	rise	written	wrote	
record	reason	rate	write			
red	reach					
rest						

/rʌ/	/raʊ/	/ræ/	/rɑ/	/rɔ/
run	around	ran	rock	wrong
rush	round			

Everyday Language

Phrases	*Sentences*
/rɛ/	
1. already did it	1. I already did it.
2. ready yet	2. Is it ready yet?
3. need a rest	3. Boy, do I need a rest!
4. the red one	4. Who's got the red one?
5. wrong direction	5. Hey, you sent me in the wrong direction!
/ri/	
1. really gone	1. He's really gone!
2. reach that high	2. I can't reach that high, can you?
3. didn't realize	3. We didn't realize you'd care so much.
4. one good reason	4. Give me one good reason and I will.
5. have to read	5. Do I have to read the whole thing?

Phrases	*Sentences*
/re/	
1. always rain	1. Why does it always rain on Monday?
2. in the race	2. I bet I can beat you in the race.
3. raise the window	3. Someone raise the window–it's hot!
4. at the railroad	4. You have to stop at the railroad.
5. think I'll rate	5. How do you think I'll rate in the contest?
/raɪ/	
1. get it right	1. Get it right this time.
2. write me	2. I wish she'd write me a letter sometime.
3. the moon rise	3. Let's go watch the moon rise.
4. arrive sometime	4. He's supposed to arrive sometime about ten o'clock.
5. ride to school	5. Do you think he'll give us a ride to school?
/rɪ/	
1. get rich	1. How can I get rich quick?
2. a ring	2. Give him a ring if you can.
3. in the river	3. Go jump in the river!
4. written in weeks	4. She hasn't written in weeks.
5. be rich	5. You have to be rich to get one.
/ro/	
1. up the road	1. Watch him tear up the road!
2. pin a rose	2. Pin a rose on me.
3. roll out	3. It's time to get up–roll out!
4. she wrote	4. Is that all she wrote?
5. cinnamon roll	5. I'll take a cinnamon roll.
/ru/	
1. know the rule	1. Come on, you know the rule.
2. fix the roof	2. You'd better fix the roof now.
3. off the roof	3. Gosh, he almost fell off the roof!
4. funny rule	4. Who made this funny rule?
5. rule him out	5. Don't rule him out just yet.
/rʌ/	
1. run me nuts	1. It's about to run me nuts!
2. run this place	2. Does she run this place?
3. the rush	3. What's the rush?
4. rush me	4. Just don't rush me!
5. on the run	5. I've been on the run all day.

Phrases	*Sentences*
/raʊ/	
1. around the block	1. Let's go two times around the block.
2. run around	2. She gave me the run around.
3. round she goes	3. Round and round she goes!
4. around your neck	4. Put it around your neck.
5. around someplace	5. It's got to be around someplace.
/ræ/	
1. ran up	1. . . . the mouse ran up the clock.
2. ran out	2. His time ran out.
3. ran me nuts	3. She almost ran me nuts!
4. ran fastest	4. She ran fastest? You're kidding!
5. ran away	5. My dog ran away–did you see him?
/rɑ/	
1. rock the boat	1. Don't rock the boat!
2. hard as a rock	2. His head is hard as a rock.
3. Rock 'N Roll	3. What happened to "Rock 'N Roll"?
4. a rock	4. We're between a rock and a hard place.
5. rock and a stone	5. Are a rock and a stone the same thing?
/rɔ/	
1. all wrong	1. You're got it all wrong.
2. wrong way	2. That's the wrong way.
3. wrong button	3. Who pushed the wrong button?
4. wrong time	4. You got it at the wrong time.
5. wrong place	5. This is the wrong place, I guess.

/r/ CONTEXTS

Distinctive features: linguaalveolar, retroflex-glide, voiced (semivowel)
/r/ ***vowel combinations:*** Initial position of an unstressed syllable

Deep Test

/rɪ/ every   /rə/ several   /ro/ railroad

Common Words

/rɪ/	/rə/	/ro/
century	natural	railroad
every	several	
everything		
receive		
refuse		
regard		
remain		
remember		
remove		
reply		
report		
require		
result		
return		
story		

Everyday Language

Phrases	*Sentences*
/rɪ/	
1. everything nice	1. He does everything nice.
2. remember the way	2. I remember the way.
3. that story	3. I told that story last.
4. please return	4. Please return to your seats.
5. every day	5. We do it every day.
/rə/	
1. natural leader	1. He's a natural leader.
2. seem natural	2. That doesn't seem natural.
3. several kids	3. Several kids flunked the test.
4. several ways	4. He knows several ways.
5. several times	5. I've gone several times.
/ro/	
1. model railroad	1. He wants a model railroad.
2. railroad tracks	2. Railroad tracks are bumpy.
3. railroad station	3. That railroad station looks dumpy.
4. by the railroad	4. Go down by the railroad.
5. old railroad	5. Old railroad engines are neat.

/r/ CONTEXTS

Distinctive features: linguaalveolar, retroflex-glide, voiced (semivowel)
/r/ ***vowel combinations:*** Final position of a stressed syllable

Deep Test

/ɛr/ bear	/ɔr/ war	/or/ four	/ær/ narrow	/aɪr/ tire	/aʊr/ hour
/ɪr/ clear	/ɑr/ car	/ʊr/ sure			

Common Words

/ɛr/	/ɪr/	/ɔr/	/ɑr/	/or/	/ʊr/
affair	appear	corner	are	before	during
air	clear	for	army	door	poor
bear	dear	foreign	article	floor	sure
care	ear	forest	car	four	you're
chair	experience	former	far	more	your
dare	fear	forward	farmer	shore	
declare	hear	important	garden	store	
fair	material	nor	market		
hair	near	or	party		
pair	nearly	order	star		
prepare	period	quarter	bar		
share	spirit	tomorrow			
square	year	war			
tear					
their					
there					
various					
very					
wear					
where					

Everyday Language

Phrases	*Sentences*
/ɛr/	
1. as a bear	1. I'm hungry as a bear!
2. funny pair	2. They make a funny pair.
3. tear me up	3. You tear me up.
4. thing to wear	4. I don't have a thing to wear.
5. as air	5. It's as thin as air.

Phrases	*Sentences*
/ɪr/	
1. clear to him	1. Make it clear to him.
2. nearly up	2. His time's nearly up.
3. the spirit	3. That's the spirit!
4. new material	4. You'll need new material.
5. no fear	5. Have no fear, _____ is here!
/ɔr/	
1. order me	1. Order me a hot dog and a coke.
2. for me	2. Get a coke for me, too.
3. a quarter	3. Can you give me a quarter?
4. back tomorrow	4. I'll pay you back tomorrow.
5. important job	5. You've got an important job.
/ɑr/	
1. new car	1. Boy, did you see his new car?
2. have a party	2. Come up. She's going to have a party.
3. joined the army	3. I think Bill joined the army.
4. big star	4. He's a big star now.
5. are you	5. Are you almost done?
/or/	
1. before you go	1. Finish before you go.
2. four times	2. I told him four times now.
3. one more	3. One more time and I quit!
4. at the door	4. Who's at the door?
5. that store	5. That store doesn't have it.
/ʊr/	
1. poor thing	1. Oh, the poor thing!
2. during school	2. They can do it during school.
3. you're not	3. You're not kidding.
4. your seat	4. Get in your seat—now!
5. sure thing	5. It looks like a sure thing.
/ær/	
1. what a character	1. What a character he is!
2. can't carry	2. You can't carry that big thing.
3. narrow gate	3. Go in the narrow gate.
4. marry me	4. Who'd want to marry me?
5. carry all	5. I can't carry all of it.

Phrases	*Sentences*
/aɪr/	
1. desire to go	1. I just have no desire to go.
2. hot as fire	2. I'm hot as fire!
3. require it	3. Why does she require it?
4. my tire	4. My tire has had it!
5. where's the fire	5. OK, buddy, where's the fire?
/aʊr/	
1. our house	1. Come to our house first.
2. noon hour	2. Let's go over the noon hour.
3. lunch hour	3. When is your lunch hour?
4. our time	4. We'll just take our time.
5. our turn	5. When is it our turn?

/r/ CONTEXTS

Distinctive features: linguaalveolar, retroflex-glide, voiced (semivowel)
/r/ ***blend combinations:*** Initial position of a stressed syllable

Deep Test

/pr/ press	/tr/ trade	/kr/ cross	/fr/ free	/spr/ spring
/br/ break	/dr/ draw	/gr/ grow	/θr/ three	/str/ strong

Common Words

/pr/	/tr/	/gr/	/br/	/dr/	/fr/	/str/
practice	control	agree	branch	draw	afraid	destroy
present	trade	degree	break	dream	free	straight
president	train	grant	bridge	dress	fresh	strange
press	travel	grass	bright	drink	friend	stream
pretty	tree	gray	bring	drive	from	street
price	tried	great	broken	drop	front	strength
prince	trip	green	brother	dry	fruit	strong
probably	trouble	grew	brought			
problem	true	ground	brown			
promise	trust	group				
proper	truth	grow				
prove	try					
surprise						

/kr/	/θr/	/spr/
across	three	spread
cross	through	spring
crowd		
cry		
increase		

Everyday Language

Phrases	***Sentences***
/pr/	
1. good price	1. That's a good price.
2. pretty nice	2. He's a pretty nice guy.
3. probably can	3. I probably can–can you?
4. surprise you	4. Did it surprise you?
5. got a problem	5. Man, you've got a problem!
/tr/	
1. trust me	1. You can trust me, can't you?
2. in trouble	2. If I do it, I'm in trouble.
3. if you try	3. You can do it if you try.
4. I tried	4. I tried and tried, but can't do it.
5. I'll trade	5. I'll trade you–even up.

Phrases	*Sentences*
/gr/	
1. great day	1. It's a great day!
2. grow up	2. Why don't you grow up?
3. paint it green	3. Paint it green or white.
4. cut the grass	4. I hate to cut the grass.
5. I agree	5. I agree, she's beautiful!
/br/	
1. Oh, brother	1. Oh, brother, not another one!
2. who brought	2. Who brought the potato chips?
3. break it	3. Don't break it—it's mine.
4. branch out	4. You should branch out if you can.
5. it's broken	5. Too bad, it's broken.
/dr/	
1. dress up	1. It's going to be a dress up dance.
2. drop it	2. Let's drop it—it's a sad subject.
3. want a drink	3. Do you want a drink?
4. you drive	4. I'll go if you drive.
5. dry your hands	5. Dry your hands on my towel.
/fr/	
1. one free	1. Buy one—get one free!
2. good friend	2. He's my good friend.
3. fresh start	3. He'll get a fresh start today.
4. from home	4. Oh boy—a note from home!
5. up front	5. It's what's up front that counts.
/str/	
1. get it straight	1. Try to get it straight this time.
2. strange way	2. That's a strange way to do it, but OK.
3. destroy me	3. You just destroy me!
4. what street	4. What street do you live on?
5. be strong	5. Be strong—it'll soon be done.
/kr/	
1. a crowd	1. Two's company—three's a crowd!
2. don't cry	2. Don't cry over spilled anything.
3. we cross	3. This is the spot we cross.
4. once across	4. Once across is enough.
5. big increase	5. That's a big increase.

Phrases	*Sentences*
/θr/	
1. three times	1. Three times three is ____.
2. about through	2. Are you just about through?
3. three wishes	3. Now–you have three wishes!
4. through and through	4. He's a Yankee through and through.
5. you're through	5. OK, friend, you're through.
/spr/	
1. spread it on	1. Peanut butter–spread it on thick!
2. spring has	2. Spring has ____.
3. spread on	3. Put the spread on top.
4. spring is	4. The spring is broken, I think.
5. til spring	5. Wait til spring when it's nice.

/r/ CONTEXTS

Distinctive features: linguaalveolar, retroflex-glide, voiced (semivowel)
/r/ ***blend combinations:*** Initial position of an unstressed syllable

Deep Test

/pr/ prepare /tr/ country /dr/ hundred

Common Words

/pr/	/tr/	/dr/
prepare	country	children
produce	history	hundred
provide	industry	

Everyday Language

Phrases	*Sentences*
/pr/	
1. provide some time	1. They'll have to provide some time.
2. prepare now	2. You need to prepare now.
3. produce the thing	3. Who'll produce the thing we need?
4. prepare to go	4. I'll prepare to go now.
5. provide it all	5. I can't provide it all the time.

/tr/

1. country 'tis	1. My country 'tis of thee . . .
2. love history	2. I love history!
3. an industry	3. Is a hot dog an industry?
4. history of	4. What's the history of this town?
5. in the country	5. He lives in the country.

/dr/

1. hundred times	1. I've told you a hundred times.
2. children can go	2. Children can go until noon.
3. a hundred miles	3. How long? About a hundred miles.
4. a hundred times	4. How many? About a hundred times.
5. a hundred people	5. Who? A hundred people.

/r/ CONTEXTS

Distinctive features: linguaalveolar, retroflex-glide, voiced (semivowel)
/r/ ***blend combinations:*** Final position of a stressed syllable

Deep Test

/rt/ art	/rm/ arm	/rk/ dark	/rn/ born	/rtʃ/ march
/rd/ board	/rs/ horse	/rθ/ North	/rdʒ/ charge	

Common Words

/rt/	/rd/	/rm/	/rs/	/rk/	/rθ/	/rn/
art	according	arm	course	dark	North	born
court	board	farm	force	mark	forth	morning
department	guard	form	horse			
heart	hard	storm				
part	regard	warm				
report	toward					
short	yard					
sort						
start						
support						

/rdʒ/	/rtʃ/
charge	march
large	

Everyday Language

Phrases	*Sentences*
/rt/	
1. work of art	1. It's a work of art.
2. short time	2. He'll be done in a short time.
3. time to start	3. It'll soon be time to start.
4. what part	4. What part do you play?
5. good report	5. You'll get a good report.
/rd/	
1. according to	1. According to the game, I'm out.
2. hard to	2. It's hard to say some things.
3. in the yard	3. We can play in the yard.
4. guard the way	4. You'll have to guard the way.
5. toward home	5. Go toward home and you'll find it.
/rm/	
1. my arm	1. My arm is too big to fit.
2. bad storm	2. That was a bad storm!
3. good form	3. _____ was in good form tonight.
4. warm night	4. It's a warm night.
5. on the farm	5. I'd like to be back on the farm.
/rs/	
1. set the course	1. Set the course and away we go!
2. a horse	2. Don't walk–get a horse!
3. force me	3. You can't force me to do it.
4. off course	4. You're way off course.
5. as a horse	5. He's big as a horse!
/rk/	
1. on your mark	1. On your mark–go!
2. in the dark	2. Don't keep me in the dark.
3. as dark as	3. It's as dark as night.
4. mark it	4. Check it, then mark it.
5. a bit dark	5. It's a bit dark, isn't it?
/rθ/	
1. up North	1. He lives up North.
2. North Pole	2. Who comes from the North Pole?
3. come forth	3. "Come forth!" said the king.
4. up North	4. Up North, down South.
5. go forth	5. "Go forth!" he shouted.

Phrases	*Sentences*
/rn/	
1. in the morning	1. I hate to get up in the morning.
2. born to sing	2. She was born to sing!
3. good morning	3. Good morning, Mrs. _____.
4. was born	4. I was born in _____.
5. top o' the morning	5. Top o' the morning to you!
/rdʒ/	
1. big charge	1. He gets a big charge out of it.
2. large size	2. Buy the large size.
3. charge it	3. Charge it, please.
4. a charge	4. Give it a charge.
5. too large	5. It's way too large.
/rtʃ/	
1. windy March	1. It's a cold and windy March.
2. forward, march	2. Now say, "Forward, March!"
3. March comes	3. March comes before _____.
4. march in	4. Just march in and tell him.
5. march, march	5. March, March! That's all we do!

/r/ CONTEXTS

Distinctive features: linguaalveolar, retroflex-glide, voiced (semivowel)
/r/ ***blend combinations:*** Final position of an unstressed syllable

Deep Test

/rt/ effort

Common Words

/rt/
effort

Everyday Language

Phrases	*Sentences*
/rt/	
1. little effort	1. It takes just a little effort.
2. your effort	2. Your effort paid off.
3. so much effort	3. It takes so much effort.
4. some effort	4. You have to exert some effort.
5. no effort	5. There's no effort in that.

/j/ CONTEXTS

Distinctive features: linguapalatal, frictionless-glide, voiced (semivowel)
/j/ ***vowel combinations:*** Initial position of a stressed syllable

Deep Test

/jɪ/ year /jɛ/ yes /jɑ/ yard /jo/ your /ju/ you /jʌ/ young

Common Words

/ju/	/jɛ/	/jɑ/	/jʌ/	/jɪ/	/jo/
use	yellow	beyond	young	year	your
you	yes	yard			
youth	yet				
union					

Everyday Language

Phrases	*Sentences*
/ju/	
1. could use	1. I could use a nap.
2. you know	2. You know how that is!
3. today's youth	3. Today's youth are bright.
4. use some	4. Can you use some money?
5. you bet	5. You bet I can!

Phrases	*Sentences*
/jɛ/	
1. oh yes	1. Oh yes, it is!
2. just yet	2. Don't look just yet.
3. yellow coat	3. My yellow coat is clean.
4. yes or no	4. Either say yes or no.
5. here yet	5. Are they here yet?
/jɑ/	
1. beyond me	1. It's beyond me!
2. beyond help	2. He's beyond help now.
3. by the yard	3. They sell it by the yard.
4. in the yard	4. They're sitting in the yard.
5. yard work	5. Yard work can be fun.
/jʌ/	
1. too young	1. She's too young for that.
2. young people	2. Young people can help.
3. young ones	3. It has three young ones.
4. young enough	4. I'm young enough to know.
5. night is young	5. The night is young yet.
/jɪ/	
1. new year	1. Have a happy new year!
2. next year	2. Wait 'til next year!
3. what year	3. What year are you in?
4. a year old	4. It's only a year old.
5. one year	5. One year seems like the other.
/jo/	
1. your name	1. What's your name?
2. your car	2. Is this your car?
3. your time	3. Your time is up.
4. your partner	4. I'm your partner.
5. your help	5. Your help is needed.

/j/ CONTEXTS

Distinctive features: linguapalatal, frictionless-glide, voiced (semivowel)
/j/ ***vowel combinations:*** Initial position of an unstressed syllable

Deep Test

/ju/ value   /jə/ million

Common Words

/ju/	/jə/
continue	million
value	union

Everyday Language

Phrases	*Sentences*
/ju/	
1. we'll continue	1. We'll continue tomorrow.
2. good value	2. That's a good value.
3. I value	3. I value your opinion.
4. continue talking	4. Continue talking while I work.
5. can't continue	5. We can't continue like this.
/jə/	
1. million dollars	1. I bet you a million dollars!
2. the union	2. Did you join the union?
3. union may	3. The union may call a strike.
4. million people	4. Over a million people watched on TV.
5. million years	5. It wouldn't happen in a million years!

/m/ CONTEXTS

Distinctive features: bilabial, nasal-continuant, voiced
/m/ ***vowel combinations:*** Initial position of a stressed syllable

Deep Test

/mi/ me	/mɛ/ met	/mɔ/ morning	/mu/ moon	/maɪ/ my
/mɪ/ miss	/mæ/ man	/mo/ most	/mʌ/ must	/maʊ/ mouth
/me/ may	/mɑ/ march			

Common Words

/mɛ/	/mɪ/	/mæ/	/mʌ/	/mi/	/mɑ/
many	admit	command	among	me	march
marry	middle	demand	money	mean	mark
measure	milk	man	month	meat	market
member	million	manner	mother	meet	modern
men	minute	master	much	meeting	tomorrow
mention	miss	matter	must		
met	permit				
method					
remember					

/maɪ/	/mu/	/me/	/maʊ/	/mo/	/mɔ/
might	moon	made	amount	moment	morning
mile	move	make	mount	more	
mind	movement	may	mountain	most	
mine	remove	remain	mouth		
my					

Everyday Language

Phrases	*Sentences*
/mɛ/	
1. how many	1. How many are there?
2. marry me	2. Will you marry me?
3. we met	3. We met last week.
4. mention it	4. Don't mention it.
5. remember to	5. Remember to call me!
/mɪ/	
1. milk and cookies	1. Want some milk and cookies?
2. wait a minute	2. Wait a minute now!
3. miss you	3. I'll miss you when you're gone.
4. get the permit	4. Did you get the permit?
5. in the middle	5. We're right in the middle.
/mæ/	
1. in command	1. Who's in command?
2. they demand	2. They demand payment first.
3. the matter	3. What's the matter with you?
4. that man	4. Who was that man?
5. master it	5. You can master it if you try.

Phrases	*Sentences*
/mʌ/	
1. among friends	1. You're among friends.
2. enough money	2. Is there enough money?
3. a month	3. A month from today we start.
4. must ask	4. You must ask first.
5. my mother	5. My mother will be here.
/mi/	
1. don't mean it	1. You don't mean it!
2. pick me	2. I hope they don't pick me.
3. get the meat	3. Did you get the meat?
4. do we meet	4. Where do we meet?
5. the meeting	5. The meeting is at seven.
/mɑ/	
1. will march	1. The band will march on Saturday.
2. have a mark	2. It doesn't have a mark on it.
3. the market	3. Let's stop at the market.
4. thoroughly modern	4. She's thoroughly modern!
5. tomorrow is	5. Tomorrow is soon enough.
/mu/	
1. moon is	1. The moon is up.
2. make a move	2. Don't make a move!
3. joined the movement	3. They joined the movement.
4. your move	4. It's your move now.
5. remove your	5. Remove your shoes before you go.
/maɪ/	
1. might be	1. He might be able to go.
2. it's a mile	2. It's a mile down the road.
3. your mind	3. Make up your mind.
4. mine is	4. Mine is already made up.
5. my, my	5. My, my, aren't you fast!
/me/	
1. made a mistake	1. You've made a mistake.
2. make me laugh	2. You make me laugh.
3. may not	3. He may not tell us.
4. that'll remain	4. That'll remain to be seen.
5. got it made	5. We've got it made now.

Phrases	*Sentences*
/maʊ/	
1. amount to much	1. It won't amount to much.
2. mount this picture	2. Can you mount this picture?
3. there's a mountain	3. There's a mountain of dishes!
4. big mouth	4. You and your big mouth!
5. mount up	5. Get ready to mount up!
/mo/	
1. wait a moment	1. Wait a moment, friends.
2. one more	2. Let's go one more round.
3. most of all	3. Most of all, it's fun.
4. take a moment	4. It'll take a moment to fix.
5. any more cake	5. Is there any more cake?
/mɔ/	
1. good morning	1. Good morning, everybody!
2. one morning	2. One morning it was just there!
3. in the morning	3. We'll start early in the morning.
4. morning is	4. Morning is my best time.
5. tomorrow morning	5. Call me tomorrow morning.

/m/ CONTEXTS

Distinctive features: bilabial, nasal-continuant, voiced
/m/ ***vowel contexts:*** Initial position of an unstressed syllable

Deep Test

/mɪ/ army /mo/ almost /mɚ/ farmer /mə/ human /maɪ/ myself

Common Words

/mə/	/mɪ/	/mɚ/	/mo/	/maɪ/
animal	army	farmer	almost	myself
department	enemy	former		
famous		summer		
gentlemen				
government				
human				
machine				
material				
moment				
movement				

Everyday Language

Phrases	*Sentences*
/mə/	
1. kind of animal	1. What kind of animal is that?
2. famous place	2. That's a famous place.
3. real gentlemen	3. He's a real gentlemen.
4. only human	4. You're only human.
5. what department	5. What department are you in?
/mɪ/	
1. in the army	1. He's in the army.
2. biggest enemy	2. She's my biggest enemy.
3. army needs	3. The army needs you.
4. made an enemy	4. You've made an enemy.
5. army food	5. You've heard about army food?
/mɚ/	
1. former mayor	1. He's the former mayor.
2. ask the farmer	2. Ask the farmer for help.
3. the former	3. Is it the former or the latter?
4. farmer in	4. Sing "Farmer in the Dell" next, please.
5. be a farmer	5. You could be a farmer.
/mo/	
1. almost ready	1. I'm almost ready.
2. almost finished	2. It's almost finished.
3. almost missed	3. You almost missed.
4. almost everyone	4. Almost everyone does.
5. almost flipped	5. I almost flipped!

Phrases	*Sentences*
/maɪ/	
1. go there myself	1. I wouldn't go there myself.
2. ask myself	2. I ask myself every day!
3. better than myself	3. Who knows better than myself?
4. myself	4. I need it myself.
5. by myself	5. I'll do it by myself.

/m/ CONTEXTS

Distinctive features: bilabial, nasal-continuant, voiced
/m/ ***vowel combinations:*** Final position of a stressed syllable

Deep Test

/im/ seem	/em/ came	/æm/ am	/um/ room	/aɪm/ time
/ɪm/ him	/ɛm/ them	/om/ home	/ʌm/ some	

Common Words

/ʌm/	/em/	/im/	/ɛm/	/ɪm/	/æm/
become	became	dream	member	him	am
come	came	seem	remember	simple	example
company	game	stream	them		
from	name				
number	same				
some					
something					
sometimes					

/om/	/um/	/aɪm/
home	room	time

Everyday Language

Phrases	*Sentences*
/ʌm/	
1. two's company	1. Two's company, three's a crowd!
2. say something	2. Say something nice.
3. sometimes I wonder	3. Sometimes I wonder about you.
4. come back	4. Come back again soon.
5. phone number	5. What's your phone number?

Phrases	*Sentences*
/em/	
1. your name	1. What's your name?
2. a fun game	2. This is a fun game.
3. all the same	3. If it's all the same with you.
4. came too late	4. We came too late.
5. same name	5. We have the same name.
/im/	
1. seem happy	1. You seem happy.
2. funny dream	2. I had a funny dream.
3. lovely stream	3. What a lovely stream!
4. seem to be	4. I seem to be wrong.
5. what they seem	5. Things aren't what they seem.
/ɛm/	
1. remember me	1. Do you remember me?
2. be a member	2. You could be a member.
3. give them	3. Give them to me.
4. hard to remember	4. It's hard to remember everything.
5. need them	5. We need them to help.
/ɪm/	
1. keep it simple	1. Keep it simple today.
2. ask him	2. Ask him for it.
3. simple person	3. I'm a simple person.
4. simple problem	4. This is a simple problem.
5. knew him	5. I knew him a little bit.
/æm/	
1. bad example	1. This is a bad example.
2. another example	2. Give another example.
3. who I am	3. Do you know who I am?
4. good example	4. Here's a good example.
5. I am	5. But I am listening!
/om/	
1. soon be home	1. We'll soon be home.
2. your home	2. Where's your home?
3. go home	3. Let's go home.
4. my home town	4. This is my home town.
5. come home	5. Come home with me.

Phrases	*Sentences*
/um/	
1. make room	1. Make room for me.
2. my room	2. Here's my room.
3. a nice room	3. Get us a nice room.
4. this room	4. This room has a view.
5. enough room	5. Is there enough room?
/aɪm/	
1. have the time	1. We have the time.
2. any time	2. Any time will do.
3. what time	3. What time is it?
4. this time	4. This time we'll do it.
5. time out	5. Time out, please.

/m/ CONTEXTS

Distinctive features: bilabial, nasal-continuant, voiced
/m/ ***vowel combinations:*** Final position of an unstressed syllable

Deep Test

/ɪm/ important /ɛm/ themselves /əm/ complete

Common Words

/əm/	/ɪm/	/ɛm/
complete	himself	themselves
problem	important	
system		

Everyday Language

Phrases	*Sentences*
/əm/	
1. complete set	1. Here's a complete set.
2. the problem	2. What's the problem?
3. know the system	3. You know the system.
4. complete it	4. When will they complete it?
5. be complete	5. When will it be complete?

Phrases	*Sentences*
/ɪm/	
1. help himself	1. Let him help himself.
2. is important	2. Look, this is important!
3. gave himself	3. He gave himself away.
4. important job	4. This is an important job.
5. so important	5. What's so important about it?
/ɛm/	
1. not themselves	1. They're not themselves tonight.
2. hate themselves	2. They'll hate themselves in the morning!
3. call themselves	3. They call themselves friends.
4. by themselves	4. Are they by themselves?
5. blame themselves	5. They can blame themselves.

/m/ CONTEXTS

Distinctive features: bilabial, nasal-continuant, voiced
/m/ ***blends:*** Final position of a stressed syllable

Deep Test

/mp/ camp   /mpt/ attempt

Common Words

/mp/	/mpt/
camp	attempt

Everyday Language

Phrases	*Sentences*
/mp/	
1. make camp	1. Let's make camp.
2. camp out	2. Do you camp out?
3. our camp	3. Our camp is nearby.
4. the camp stove	4. Where's the camp stove?
5. we'll camp	5. We'll camp over night.

Phrases	*Sentences*
/mpt/	
1. attempt it	1. I wouldn't attempt it.
2. second attempt	2. It's his second attempt.
3. attempt anything	3. She'll attempt anything.
4. could attempt	4. We could attempt it.
5. last attempt	5. Our last attempt failed.

/m/ CONTEXTS

Distinctive features: bilabial, nasal-continuant, voiced
/m/ ***blends:*** Final position of an unstressed syllable

Deep Test

/mz/ sometimes

Common Words

/mz/

sometimes

Everyday Language

Phrases	*Sentences*
/mz/	
1. sometimes I'm	1. Sometimes I'm happy.
2. kill me sometimes	2. You just kill me sometimes!
3. go there sometimes	3. They go there sometimes.
4. sometimes I	4. Sometimes I doubt it.
5. sometimes it	5. Sometimes it seems hopeless.

/n/ CONTEXTS

Distinctive features: linguaalveolar, nasal-continuant, voiced
/n/ ***vowel combinations:*** Initial position of a stressed syllable

Deep Test

/ni/ knee	/nɛ/ neck	/nɔ/ north	/nu/ new	/naɪ/ nice
/nɪ/ near	/næ/ national	/no/ no	/nʌ/ none	/naʊ/ now
/ne/ name	/nɑ/ not			

Common Words

/ne/	/no/	/nɛ/	/nu/	/nʌ/	/naɪ/
name	know	narrow	afternoon	another	knight
nation	known	necessary	knew	enough	nice
native	no	neck	new	none	nine
nature	nose	never	news	nothing	
neighbor	note	next	newspaper	number	
	notice				

/ni/	/nɪ/	/næ/	/nɑ/	/nɔ/	/naʊ/
knee	near	national	knowledge	north	now
need	nearly	natural	not		
neither					

Everyday Language

Phrases	***Sentences***
/ne/	
1. her name	1. Get her name!
2. my neighbor	2. She's my neighbor.
3. native state	3. What's your native state?
4. nature stories	4. I love nature stories.
5. great nation	5. This is a great nation.
/no/	
1. know better	1. I know better now.
2. still no	2. The answer is still no.
3. my nose	3. My nose feels funny.
4. notice her	4. Did you notice her hair?
5. known each other	5. They've known each other awhile.

Phrases	*Sentences*
/nɛ/	
1. narrow escape	1. That was a narrow escape!
2. really necessary	2. Is it really necessary?
3. fool neck	3. You'll break your fool neck!
4. never said	4. I never said that.
5. next time	5. Just wait 'til next time!
/nu/	
1. this afternoon	1. Try again this afternoon.
2. you knew	2. You knew that would happen.
3. new car	3. See my new car?
4. any news	4. Is there any news?
5. the newspaper	5. She works for the newspaper.
/nʌ/	
1. another story	1. That's another story.
2. had enough	2. Have you had enough?
3. none of them	3. None of them came.
4. knows nothing	4. She knows nothing about it.
5. what number	5. What number do you have?
/naɪ/	
1. knight in armor	1. He's a knight in shining armor!
2. will be nice	2. That will be nice.
3. nine lives	3. Does a cat really have nine lives?
4. nice day	4. Have a nice day!
5. you're nice	5. You're nice to say that.
/ni/	
1. my knee	1. I hurt my knee.
2. bended knee	2. Say it on bended knee.
3. you need	3. You need a doctor.
4. we need	4. We need to talk about it.
5. bend your knee	5. Bend your knee a little.
/nɪ/	
1. nearly five	1. It's nearly five o'clock.
2. is near	2. That time of year is near.
3. nearly hit us	3. They nearly hit us!
4. nowhere near	4. We've nowhere near our goal.
5. near miss	5. That was a near miss.

Phrases	*Sentences*
/næ/	
1. national disaster	1. It's a national disaster!
2. natural foods	2. Natural foods are best.
3. only natural	3. It's only natural.
4. natural lake	4. This is a natural lake.
5. national figure	5. He's a national figure.
/nɑ/	
1. my knowledge	1. My knowledge is limited.
2. that's not	2. That's not what I hear.
3. little knowledge	3. A little knowledge helps.
4. some knowledge	4. Some knowledge is dangerous.
5. not kidding	5. You're not kidding!
/nɔ/	
1. north wind	1. It's a north wind.
2. mile north	2. Go a mile north.
3. face north	3. Face north now.
4. north side	4. Look on the north side.
5. up north	5. Let's move up north.
/naʊ/	
1. now you're	1. Now you're talking!
2. now is	2. Now is a good time.
3. wrong now	3. What's wrong now?
4. now you	4. Now you tell me!
5. you're now	5. You're now the boss.

/n/ CONTEXTS

Distinctive features: linguaalveolar, nasal-continuant, voiced
/n/ ***vowel combinations:*** Initial position of an unstressed syllable

Deep Test

/nɪ/ evening /nə/ journal /nɚ/ corner

Common Words

/nɪ/	/nə/	/nɚ/
any	animal	corner
anything	finally	dinner
business	general	honor
company	journal	manner
evening	minute	
finish		
many		
money		
morning		

Everyday Language

Phrases	*Sentences*
/nɪ/	
1. funny business	1. Looks like funny business.
2. having company	2. Are we having company?
3. this evening	3. Come this evening.
4. in the morning	4. See you in the morning.
5. down to business	5. Let's get down to business.
/nə/	
1. finally we	1. Finally we can go.
2. journal came	2. The journal came today.
3. strange animal	3. That's a strange animal.
4. general rule	4. That's the general rule.
5. a minute	5. Wait a minute!
/nɚ/	
1. around the corner	1. It's just around the corner.
2. to dinner	2. Can you come to dinner tonight?
3. this corner	3. Fold this corner down.
4. your honor	4. It's in your honor.
5. nice manner	5. He has a nice manner.

/n/ CONTEXTS

Distinctive features: linguaalveolar, nasal-continuant, voiced
/n/ ***vowel combinations:*** Final position of a stressed syllable

Deep Test

/in/ seen	/ɛn/ ten	/ɔn/ on	/un/ moon	/ʌn/ sun	/aʊn/ down
/ɪn/ in	/æn/ an	/on/ own	/ɝn/ turn	/aɪn/ fine	/ɔɪn/ join
/en/ gain					

Common Words

/ɛn/	/ɪn/	/ʌn/	/en/	/æn/	/in/
again	begin	country	contain	an	between
attention	continue	done	danger	answer	clean
been	in	hundred	explain	began	green
center	industry	none	gain	can	machine
century	interest	one	obtain	man	mean
enemy	into	run	pain	plan	queen
enter	opinion	son	plain	ran	scene
gentle	skin	sun	rain	than	seen
gentleman	thin	under	remain		
men	win	wonder			
mention	window	wonderful			
ten	winter				
then	within				
twenty					
when					

/aɪn/	/on/	/un/	/ɝn/	/aʊn/	/ɔn/	/ɔɪn/
fine	alone	afternoon	burn	brown	gone	join
line	known	moon	learn	down	on	
mile	only	soon	return	mountain	upon	
mine	own	union	turn	town		
nine	stone					
sign						

Everyday Language

Phrases	*Sentences*
/ɛn/	
1. go again	1. It's time to go again.
2. do not enter	2. The sign says Do Not Enter.
3. it's been	3. It's been a long time.
4. off center	4. He's a little off center.
5. be gentle	5. Be gentle with it.
/ɪn/	
1. can't begin	1. I can't begin to tell you . . .
2. the window	2. Open the window.
3. cold winter	3. It's been a cold winter.
4. your skin	4. Your skin looks red.
5. so thin	5. You've gotten so thin!
/ʌn/	
1. finally done	1. Well, that's finally done.
2. in the country	2. Do you live in the country?
3. run over	3. Run over there for me.
4. your son	4. Can your son go along?
5. wonder where	5. I wonder where she is?
/en/	
1. to explain	1. Don't try to explain.
2. like rain	2. It looks like rain.
3. plain truth	3. The plain truth will do.
4. in pain	4. Are you in pain?
5. contain sugar	5. Does this contain sugar?
/æn/	
1. they began	1. They began too late.
2. your plan	2. What's your plan?
3. can I	3. Can I be of help?
4. more than	4. We need you more than you know.
5. right answer	5. Who has the right answer?
/in/	
1. between the lines	1. You must read between the lines.
2. green one	2. My green one will fit you.
3. do you mean	3. What do you mean?
4. like a queen	4. She looks like a queen!
5. bad scene	5. That's a bad scene!

Phrases	*Sentences*
/aɪn/	
1. just fine	1. That's just fine!
2. on the line	2. Stay on the line.
3. use mine	3. You may use mine.
4. for the sign	4. Look for the sign.
5. nine of us	5. There'll be nine of us.
/on/	
1. go alone	1. Plan to go alone.
2. only have	2. You only have five minutes.
3. own one	3. He doesn't own one.
4. as stone	4. It's hard as stone.
5. not known	5. That's probably not known.
/un/	
1. for the moon	1. Watch for the moon.
2. up soon	2. It'll be up soon.
3. all afternoon	3. I slept all afternoon.
4. union meets	4. The union meets tonight.
5. soon tell	5. I can soon tell you.
/ɝn/	
1. bad burn	1. That's a bad burn
2. learn how	2. You must learn how.
3. return the book	3. Return the book today.
4. turn around	4. Turn around slowly.
5. burn yourself	5. Don't burn yourself!
/aʊn/	
1. paint it brown	1. Just paint it brown to match.
2. come down	2. Come down this instant!
3. climbing a mountain	3. It's like climbing a mountain.
4. in town	4. Were you in town?
5. brown bag	5. Do you have a brown bag?
/ɔn/	
1. all gone	1. Well, it's all gone.
2. upon a time	2. Once upon a time . . .
3. turn on	3. Turn on the stove.
4. gone today	4. They're gone today.
5. on your side	5. I'm on your side.

Phrases	*Sentences*
/ɔɪn/	
1. join us	1. Come join us.
2. join together	2. They join together here.
3. join 'em	3. If you can't beat 'em, join 'em!
4. join the crowd	4. Join the crowd, my friend!
5. join up	5. We'll join up later.

/n/ CONTEXTS

Distinctive features: linguaalveolar, nasal-continuant, voiced
/n/ ***vowel combinations:*** Final position of an unstressed syllable

Deep Test

/ɪn/ indeed /ən/ common /ɚn/ modern

Common Words

/ən/	/ɪn/	/ɚn/
action	captain	modern
attention	children	
common	enjoy	
condition	even	
consider	foreign	
contain	given	
continue	happen	
control	heaven	
direction	human	
gentleman	include	
iron	increase	
mention	indeed	
million	instead	
nation	kitchen	
natural	often	
ocean	open	
opinion	taken	
position	women	
question		
seven		
station		
understand		
union		
unless		
until		
woman		

Everyday Language

Phrases	*Sentences*
/ən/	
1. little action	1. Let's get a little action here!
2. consider going	2. Would you consider going?
3. don't mention	3. Don't mention her name.
4. hard question	4. That's a hard question.
5. lost control	5. They surely lost control.
/ɪn/	
1. enjoy opera	1. Do you enjoy opera?
2. didn't even	2. He didn't even say "thanks."
3. what will happen	3. I don't know what will happen.
4. include the tax	4. Does that include the tax?
5. in the kitchen	5. Let's sit in the kitchen.
/ɚn/	
1. modern sound	1. That's a modern sound.
2. modern way	2. This is the modern way.
3. very modern	3. It's not very modern
4. he's modern	4. He's modern in his dress.
5. modern housing	5. Modern housing is scarce.

/n/ CONTEXTS

Distinctive features: linguaalveolar, nasal-continuant, voiced
/n/ ***blends:*** Final position of a stressed syllable

Deep Test

/nt/ account /nd/ and /ns/ chance /nst/ against /ntʃ/ branch

Common Words

/nd/	/nt/	/ns/	/ntʃ/	/nst/
and	account	advance	branch	against
around	amount	chance	inch	
behind	can't	dance		
beyond	cent	once		
command	count	prince		
demand	don't	sense		
end	front	since		
find	grant			
found	mount			
friend	paint			
ground	plant			
kind	point			
land	sent			
mind	want			
pound	went			
round	won't			
send				
sound				
spend				
stand				
understand				
wind				

Everyday Language

Phrases	*Sentences*
/nd/	
1. you and me	1. It's just you and me.
2. near the end	2. We're near the end now.
3. kind of pie	3. What kind of pie do you have?
4. stand there	4. Don't just stand there!
5. find it	5. Where did you find it?
/nt/	
1. my account	1. My account is overdrawn.
2. get a cent	2. You won't get a cent!
3. count on anything	3. Don't count on anything.
4. paint that	4. Did you paint that?
5. up front	5. Let's sit up front.

Phrases	*Sentences*
/ns/	
1. to the dance	1. Are you going to the dance?
2. once in awhile	2. Once in awhile I do.
3. no sense	3. There's no sense stopping.
4. since when	4. Since when did they start that?
5. he's a prince	5. He's a prince of a guy!
/ntʃ/	
1. which branch	1. Which branch do you use?
2. inch short	2. It's an inch short.
3. grew an inch	3. He just grew an inch.
4. that branch	4. Watch that branch!
5. lower branch	5. Chop off the lower branch.
/nst/	
1. against me	1. You're all against me!
2. against the wall	2. Stand against the wall.
3. against the post	3. Lean it against the post.
4. against smoking	4. We're against smoking.
5. they're against	5. They're against all of us.

/n/ CONTEXTS

Distinctive features: linguaalveolar, nasal-continuant, voiced
/n/ ***blends:*** Final position of an unstressed syllable

Deep Test

/nt/ department /ns/ silence /nd/ island

Common Words

/nt/	/ns/	/nd/
department	difference	husband
different	distance	island
government	experience	
important	silence	
moment		
movement		

Everyday Language

Phrases	*Sentences*
/nt/	
1. look different	1. You look different today.
2. very important	2. But it's very important!
3. moment to moment	3. From moment to moment it changes.
4. a new movement	4. They put in a new movement.
5. fire department	5. Call the fire department!
/ns/	
1. the difference	1. What's the difference?
2. no experience	2. You have no experience.
3. perfect silence	3. We'll need perfect silence.
4. long distance	4. He's calling long distance.
5. what a difference	5. What a difference a day makes!
/nd/	
1. on the island	1. We lived on the island.
2. your husband	2. Is that your husband?
3. my husband	3. My husband wouldn't like it.
4. to the island	4. Take the ferry to the island.
5. need a husband	5. You need a husband.

/ŋ/ CONTEXTS

Distinctive features: linguavelar, nasal-continuant, voiced
/ŋ/ ***vowel combinations:*** Final position of a stressed syllable

Deep Test

/ɪŋ/ king   /æŋ/ hang   /ɔŋ/ long   /ʌŋ/ among

Common Words

/ɪŋ/	/ɔŋ/	/ʌŋ/	/æŋ/
bring	along	among	hang
finger	belong	young	
king	long	uncle	
ring	song		
sing	strong		
single	wrong		
spring			
wing			

Everyday Language

Phrases	*Sentences*
/ɪŋ/	
1. bring it	1. Bring it inside.
2. put your finger	2. Put your finger in here.
3. phone ring	3. Did the phone ring?
4. single one	4. There isn't a single one left.
5. be king	5. I wonder who'll be king?
/ɔŋ/	
1. a long sad	1. It's a long, sad story!
2. be strong	2. Be strong, now!
3. what's wrong	3. What's wrong with that?
4. belong here	4. You don't belong here.
5. our song	5. They're playing our song!
/ʌŋ/	
1. among old friends	1. We're among old friends.
2. too young	2. You're too young now.
3. young man	3. When I was a young man . . .
4. still young	4. He's still young, you know.
5. monkey's uncle	5. Well, I'll be a monkey's uncle!
/æŋ/	
1. hang you	1. They can't hang you for that.
2. hang your	2. Hang your coat here.
3. doesn't hang	3. It doesn't hang straight.
4. hang of it	4. You'll get the hang of it.
5. hang up	5. Hang up your clothes, please.

/ŋ/ CONTEXTS

Distinctive features: linguavelar, nasal-continuant, voiced
/ŋ/ vowel combinations: Final position of an unstressed syllable

Deep Test

/ɪŋ/ coming

Common Words

/ɪŋ/

according
anything
being
building
coming
during
evening
everything
following
going
meeting
morning
nothing
something
thing

Everyday Language

Phrases

/ɪŋ/

1. according to
2. being funny
3. you coming
4. everything looks
5. we're going

Sentences

1. According to this, we won.
2. You're just being funny.
3. Are you coming or not?
4. Everything looks good to me.
5. We're going a little later.

/ŋ/ CONTEXTS

Distinctive features: linguavelar, nasal-continuant, voiced
/ŋ/ ***blends:*** Final position of a stressed syllable

Deep Test

/ŋk/ bank

Common Words

/ŋk/

bank
drink
thank
think

Everyday Language

Phrases	*Sentences*
/ŋk/	
1. bank opened	1. The bank opened at nine.
2. get a drink	2. Let's get a drink.
3. thank you	3. Thank you for your help.
4. I think	4. I think you're cute!
5. on the bank	5. We just sat on the bank.

/tʃ/ CONTEXTS

Distinctive features: linguaalveolar, affricative, voiceless
/tʃ/ ***vowel combinations:*** Initial position of a stressed syllable

Deep Test

/tʃi/ chief	/tʃe/ change	/tʃæ/ chance	/tʃɝ/ church
/tʃɪ/ children	/tʃɛ/ check	/tʃɑ/ charge	/tʃaɪ/ child

Common Words

/tʃɛ/	/tʃæ/	/tʃe/	/tʃɑ/	/tʃi/	/tʃaɪ/	/tʃɪ/
chair	chance	change	charge	chief	child	children
check						

/tʃɝ/
church

Everyday Language

Phrases	*Sentences*
/tʃɛ/	
1. your chair	1. Give her your chair.
2. check on	2. Check on the tickets.
3. chair back	3. Push your chair back.
4. a check	4. Just write a check.
5. check bounce	5. Did the check bounce?
/tʃæ/	
1. take a chance	1. Don't take a chance.
2. good chance	2. There's a good chance.
3. one chance	3. There's one chance in a hundred.
4. chance is	4. Chance is like fate.
5. no chance	5. There's no chance of going now.
/tʃe/	
1. change your mind	1. Maybe you'll change your mind.
2. change now	2. I have to change now.
3. movie change	3. When does the movie change?
4. change for a ten	4. Do you have change for a ten?
5. change the tire	5. I can change the tire.
/tʃɑ/	
1. in charge	1. Who's in charge?
2. charge it	2. Charge it to my account.
3. charge too much	3. They charge too much.
4. charge him	4. They'll charge him with theft.
5. charge a dollar	5. He'll only charge a dollar.

Phrases	*Sentences*
/tʃi/	
1. the chief	1. Here comes the chief.
2. chief cook	2. He's the chief cook.
3. one chief	3. One chief is enough.
4. make him chief	4. They'll make him chief.
5. chief complaint	5. My chief complaint is this.
/tʃaɪ/	
1. like a child	1. She acts like a child.
2. child's play	2. This is child's play.
3. child size	3. This is child size.
4. one more child	4. We can take one more child.
5. such a child	5. Don't be such a child.
/tʃɪ/	
1. come children	1. Come, children, time for bed.
2. children will	2. The children will be here soon.
3. for children	3. Is that safe for children?
4. will be children	4. Children will be children!
5. children aren't	5. Children aren't allowed.
/tʃɝ/	
1. time for church	1. It's time for church.
2. church bells	2. The church bells are ringing.
3. which church	3. Which church do you attend?
4. church supper	4. Are you going to the church supper?
5. church is	5. Church is after Sunday School.

/tʃ/ CONTEXTS

Distinctive features: linguaalveolar, affricative, voiceless
/tʃ/ ***vowel combinations:*** Initial position of an unstressed syllable

Deep Test

/tʃə/ question   /tʃɚ/ picture

Common Words

/tʃə/	/tʃɚ/
century	nature
question	picture

Everyday Language

Phrases	*Sentences*
/tʃə/	
1. make a century	1. A hundred years make a century.
2. good question	2. That's a good question.
3. have a question	3. Do you have a question?
4. the 19th century	4. That was in the 19th century.
5. don't question	5. Don't question his choice.
/tʃɚ/	
1. mother nature	1. Mother nature will do it.
2. picture that	2. Can you picture that?
3. get a picture	3. We want to get a picture.
4. quiet nature	4. He has a quiet nature.
5. get the picture	5. Do you get the picture?

/tʃ/ CONTEXTS

Distinctive features: linguaalveolar, affricative, voiceless
/tʃ/ **vowel *combinations:*** Final position of a stressed syllable

Deep Test

/itʃ/ each /ætʃ/ catch /ɑtʃ/ watch /ɝtʃ/ church /ʌtʃ/ much
/ɪtʃ/ rich

Common Words

/itʃ/	/ɪtʃ/	/ʌtʃ/	/ætʃ/	/ɝtʃ/	/ɑtʃ/
each	kitchen	much	catch	church	watch
reach	rich	such	natural		
speech	which	touch			
teach					
teacher					

Everyday Language

Phrases	*Sentences*
/itʃ/	
1. each person	1. Give one to each person.
2. reach it	2. Can you reach it?
3. his speech	3. His speech is better.
4. can't teach	4. You can't teach him anything.
5. your teacher	5. Where's your teacher?
/ɪtʃ/	
1. in the kitchen	1. He works in the kitchen.
2. get rich	2. He won't get rich there.
3. which place	3. Which placc is it?
4. rich people	4. Rich people work hard, too.
5. kitchen help	5. Kitchen help is hard to find.
/ʌtʃ/	
1. very much	1. I don't like that very much.
2. such a waste	2. Such a waste, it seems.
3. touch it	3. Just touch it gently.
4. much more	4. Is there much more?
5. such a mess	5. I've never seen such a mess!
/ætʃ/	
1. catch cold	1. You'll catch cold.
2. natural curl	2. Her hair has a natural curl.
3. catch the dickens	3. We may catch the dickens!
4. natural foods	4. Natural foods taste good.
5. catch anything	5. Did they catch anything?
/ɝtʃ/	
1. in church	1. They were married in church.
2. at church	2. I saw her at church.
3. church begins	3. Church begins at 11.
4. church choir	4. He sings in the church choir.
5. support the church	5. We should support the church.
/ɑtʃ/	
1. better watch	1. Better watch your step.
2. new watch	2. That's a new watch.
3. watch awhile	3. I'll just watch awhile.
4. can watch	4. You can watch the whole thing.
5. watch out	5. Watch out, clumsy!

/dʒ/ CONTEXTS

Distinctive features: linguaalveolar, affricative, voiced
/dʒ/ ***vowel combinations:*** Initial position of a stressed syllable

Deep Test

/dʒɛ/ general   /dʒɑ/ job   /dʒʌ/ just   /dʒɝ/ journal   /dʒɔɪ/ joy

Common Words

/dʒɛ/	/dʒɔɪ/	/dʒʌ/	/dʒɑ/	/dʒɝ/
general	enjoy	judge	job	journal
gentle	join	just		
gentleman	joy			
object				
suggest				

Everyday Language

Phrases	*Sentences*
/dʒɛ/	
1. general rule	1. As a general rule, no.
2. be gentle	2. Be gentle with it.
3. like a gentleman	3. You must act like a gentleman.
4. don't object	4. I don't object to that.
5. you suggest	5. What would you suggest?
/dʒɔɪ/	
1. enjoy a swim	1. Would you enjoy a swim?
2. join now	2. Better join now while you can.
3. jumped for joy	3. I nearly jumped for joy.
4. enjoy yourself	4. Try to enjoy yourself.
5. join you	5. We'll join you later.
/dʒʌ/	
1. judge for youself	1. You must judge for yourself.
2. just about	2. We're just about done.
3. just one	3. Just one more time.
4. eat just one	4. Bet you can't eat just one!
5. best judge	5. Who's the best judge of that?

Phrases	*Sentences*
/dʒa/	
1. a good job	1. That was a good job.
2. get the job	2. Did he get the job?
3. my job	3. My job is boring.
4. good job is	4. A good job is hard to find.
5. another job	5. You can always get another job.
/dʒɝ/	
1. for the journal	1. He writes for the *Journal.*
2. new journal	2. Has the new journal come?
3. in the journal	3. It's listed in the journal.
4. misplaced the journal	4. I've misplaced the journal.
5. journal article	5. It's in a recent journal article.

/dʒ/ CONTEXTS

Distinctive features: linguaalveolar, affricative, voiced
/dʒ/ ***vowel combinations:*** Initial position of an unstressed syllable

Deep Test

/dʒɛ/ subject /dʒɚ/ danger

Common Words

/dʒɚ/	/dʒɛ/
danger	subject
soldier	

Everyday Language

Phrases	*Sentences*
/dʒɚ/	
1. little danger	1. There's little danger there.
2. soldier now	2. He's a soldier now.
3. the danger sign	3. Did you see the danger sign?
4. danger was	4. Danger was everywhere!
5. that soldier	5. Let's ask that soldier.

Phrases	*Sentences*
/dʒɛ/	
1. deep subject	1. That's a deep subject!
2. subject to that	2. We're not subject to that.
3. next subject	3. What's the next subject?
4. subject to	4. Are you subject to colds?
5. drop the subject	5. Let's just drop the subject!

/dʒ/ CONTEXTS

Distinctive features: linguaalveolar, affricative, voiced
/dʒ/ ***vowel combinations:*** Final position of a stressed syllable

Deep Test

/ɪdʒ/ bridge /edʒ/ age /ɛdʒ/ edge /ʌdʒ/ judge

Common Words

/edʒ/	/ɪdʒ/	/ɛdʒ/	/ʌdʒ/
age	bridge	edge	judge
page			

Everyday Language

Phrases	*Sentences*
/edʒ/	
1. what age	1. What age are you?
2. legal age	2. Are you of legal age?
3. next page	3. Go to the next page.
4. one page	4. Just do one page at a time.
5. age a little	5. Let it age a little.
/ɪdʒ/	
1. that bridge	1. That bridge is closed.
2. toll bridge	2. We'll have to use the toll bridge.
3. new bridge	3. They're building a new bridge.
4. bridge the gap	4. It will bridge the gap.
5. raise the bridge	5. Raise the bridge, we're coming through!

Phrases	*Sentences*
/ɛdʒ/	
1. sharp edge	1. Watch that sharp edge!
2. near the edge	2. Put it near the edge.
3. keep the edge	3. Keep the edge straight.
4. straight edge	4. Who has the straight edge?
5. one edge	5. One edge is crooked.
/ʌdʒ/	
1. fair judge	1. He's a fair judge.
2. don't judge	2. Don't judge too quickly.
3. judge not	3. "Judge not, lest . . ."
4. poor judge	4. I'm a poor judge of music.
5. can't judge	5. You can't judge by that.

/dʒ/ CONTEXTS

Distinctive features: linguaalveolar, affricative, voiced
/dʒ/ ***vowel combinations:*** Final position of an unstressed syllable

Deep Test

/ɪdʒ/ passage

Common Words

/ɪdʒ/
college
knowledge
passage
village

Everyday Language

Phrases	*Sentences*
/ɪdʒ/	
1. off to college	1. He's off to college now.
2. speaking knowledge	2. She has a speaking knowledge of French.
3. last passage	3. Read the last passage.
4. tiny village	4. Oh, it's just a tiny village.
5. college education	5. You can't beat a college education.

VOWELS

/i/ CONTEXTS

Distinctive features: high-front, tense, unround
/i/ ***consonant combinations:*** Initial position of a stressed syllable

Deep Test

/i/ either /it/ eat /iv/ even /iz/ easy /itʃ/ each /ist/ east

Common Words

/i/	/it/	/iv/	/iz/	/itʃ/	/ist/
either	eat	even	easy	each	east
evening					

Everyday Language

Phrases	***Sentences***
/i/	
1. either we go	1. Either we go or we stay.
2. either left or right	2. We turn either left or right.
3. either way	3. Either way is OK.
4. like it either	4. I don't like it either.
5. in the evening	5. When? In the evening.
/it/	
1. to eat	1. What's to eat?
2. you eat	2. Did you eat yet?
3. let's eat	3. Let's eat lunch together.
4. bite to eat	4. Want to get a bite to eat?
5. ready to eat	5. We're ready to eat–c'mon!
/iv/	
1. even up	1. Let's even up sides.
2. even I can	2. Even I can do that.
3. even I know	3. Even I know how.
4. not very even	4. That's not very even–turn it.
5. even or odd	5. Is it even or odd this week?

Phrases	*Sentences*
/iz/	
1. that's easy	1. That's easy to say—hard to do.
2. no easy way	2. There's no easy way to get it done.
3. easy to do	3. Some things are easy to do.
4. easy on	4. Easy on—easy off!
5. easy does it	5. Easy does it—take your time.
/itʃ/	
1. each one	1. Each one gets a turn.
2. each and every one	2. Each and every one of you can _____.
3. each idea	3. I remember each idea.
4. each kid	4. He gave each kid a balloon.
5. each time	5. I like it better each time I go.
/ist/	
1. east is east	1. East is east and _____.
2. east of me	2. He lives east of me.
3. east coast	3. We flew to the east coast.
4. East Main	4. Her house is on East Main.
5. in the east	5. Wind in the east—fish bite least!

/i/ CONTEXTS

Distinctive features: high-front, tense, unround
/i/ ***consonant combinations:*** Medial position of a stressed syllable

Deep Test

/si/ receive	/ti/ teach	/bi/ beat	/ni/ need	/kri/ increase
/li/ believe	/hi/ heat	/ki/ keep	/wi/ week	/kwi/ queen
/mi/ mean	/ri/ reach	/ði/ these	/twi/ between	/gri/ green
/di/ deal	/pli/ complete	/ʃi/ machine	/dri/ dream	/sli/ sleep
/fi/ feel	/spi/ speech	/tʃi/ chief	/kli/ clean	/swi/ sweet
/pi/ peach	/stri/ stream			

Common Words

/si/	/li/	/mi/	/di/	/fi/	/pi/	/ti/
receive	believe	mean	deal	feel	peace	teach
scene	lead	meat	deep	feet	piece	teacher
seat	leader	meet	indeed	field		
seek	least	meeting				
seem	leave					
seen						

/hi/	/ri/	/pli/	/spi/	/stri/	/bi/	/ki/	/ði/
he's	reach	complete	speak	stream	beat	keep	these
heat	read	please	speech	street			

/ʃi/	/tʃi/	/ni/	/wi/	/twi/	/dri/	/kli/
machine	chief	need	week	between	dream	clean

/kri/	/kwi/	/gri/	/sli/	/swi/
increase	queen	green	sleep	sweet

Everyday Language

Phrases	*Sentences*
/si/	
1. your seat	1. Take your seat now.
2. seen this	2. Have you seen this?
3. seem tired	3. You seem tired today.
4. give than receive	4. It's better to give than to receive.
5. hide and seek	5. Let's play hide and seek.
/li/	
1. the leader	1. I'm the leader this time.
2. leave it alone	2. Leave it alone and see what happens.
3. lead the way	3. You're the boss, so lead the way.
4. believe you	4. I believe you can do anything.
5. my least favorite	5. Vanilla is my least favorite.
/mi/	
1. mean it	1. I didn't mean it.
2. the meat	2. Pass the meat, please.
3. to meet you	3. I'm very glad to meet you.
4. the meeting	4. Where's the meeting today?
5. meat and potatoes	5. I really like meat and potatoes.

Phrases	*Sentences*
/di/	
1. make a deal	1. Let's make a deal.
2. the cards	2. Deal the cards.
3. deep trouble	3. You're in deep trouble.
4. deep in the mud	4. He's stuck deep in the mud.
5. big deal	5. That's no big deal.
/fi/	
1. feel so good	1. I don't feel so good.
2. sore feet	2. He has sore feet.
3. left field	3. He plays left field.
4. feel great	4. I feel great!
5. six feet	5. He's over six feet tall.
/pi/	
1. piece of pie	1. Have a piece of pie.
2. Peace	2. Peace, brother.
3. world peace	3. Can we hope for world peace?
4. which piece	4. Which piece do you want?
5. each piece	5. Each piece looks good.
/ti/	
1. didn't teach	1. He didn't teach me much.
2. my teacher	2. Ms. _____ is my teacher.
3. your teacher	3. Does your teacher like to _____?
4. teach me	4. Will you teach me to do that?
5. your teacher	5. Who's your teacher for music?
/hi/	
1. he's the	1. He's the biggest _____.
2. he's the	2. He's the littlest _____.
3. he's the	3. He's the smartest _____.
4. stand the heat	4. I can't stand the heat.
5. the heat	5. Turn up the heat–it's cold.
/ri/	
1. to read books	1. I like to read books.
2. read the assignment	2. Did you read the assignment?
3. reach the top	3. Can you reach the top?
4. reach your goal	4. Did you reach your goal?
5. read a good book	5. It's a day to read a good book.

Phrases	*Sentences*
/pli/	
1. the complete story	1. I read the complete story.
2. please pass	2. Please pass the potatoes.
3. complete the project	3. Did he complete the project?
4. please show	4. Please show me how.
5. please show her	5. Please show her the way.
/spi/	
1. a speech	1. He gave a speech.
2. speak about	2. What did he speak about?
3. speech about	3. It was a speech about cars.
4. good speech	4. Was it a good speech?
5. his speech	5. His speech was great!
/stri/	
1. in the stream	1. Are there fish in the stream?
2. down the street	2. It's just down the street.
3. the street	3. They're fixing the street.
4. on the street	4. Can bikes go on the street?
5. the stream	5. The stream goes to the lake.
/bi/	
1. beat her	1. He really tried to beat her.
2. want to beat	2. Why did he want to beat her?
3. she beat	3. Because she beat him first.
4. beat him	4. Why did she beat him?
5. beat everybody	5. She can beat everybody!
/ki/	
1. keep good time	1. Those watches keep good time.
2. can I keep	2. Can I keep the prize?
3. may keep	3. You may keep the whistle.
4. do you keep	4. Where do you keep the toys?
5. keep the peace	5. Mom tried to keep peace.
/ði/	
1. are these	1. Are these your friends?
2. these aren't	2. These aren't my friends.
3. these go	3. Where do these go?
4. do these go	4. Do these go in here?
5. are these	5. Are these expensive?

Phrases	*Sentences*
/ʃi/	
1. washing machine	1. The washing machine is broken.
2. can the machine	2. Can the machine be fixed?
3. that machine	3. That machine is old.
4. a machine	4. Is a car a machine?
5. which machine	5. Which machine do you use?
/tʃi/	
1. the chief	1. Where's the chief?
2. chief of police	2. He's the chief of police.
3. fire chief	3. I want to be a fire chief.
4. chief complaint	4. What's your chief complaint?
5. be the chief	5. Someone has to be the chief.
/ni/	
1. you need	1. What do you need?
2. need a glove	2. I need a glove.
3. do you need	3. Why do you need a glove?
4. need it	4. I need it for the ballgame.
5. you need it	5. When do you need it?
/wi/	
1. next week	1. I need it next week.
2. first of next week	2. Do you want it the first of next week?
3. week from today	3. A week from today–Thursday.
4. make a week	4. Seven days make a week.
5. week overdue	5. That book's a week overdue.
/twi/	
1. between parked cars	1. Don't walk between parked cars.
2. between the lines	2. You have to read between the lines.
3. between two thorns	3. A rose between two thorns . . .
4. between the devil	4. Between the devil and the deep blue sea!
5. between the two	5. That's just between the two of you.
/dri/	
1. did you dream	1. What did you dream up?
2. my dream	2. That's my dream car.
3. dream every night	3. It seems I dream every night.
4. your dream	4. Is your dream good or bad?
5. that dream	5. I've had that dream before.

Phrases	*Sentences*
/kli/	
1. clean up	1. Clean up your room!
2. clean fish	2. Who likes to clean fish?
3. clean now	3. Are my hands clean now?
4. clean the car	4. I need to clean the car.
5. clean plate	5. See my clean plate?
/kri/	
1. price increase	1. That's a big price increase.
2. the increase	2. How much was the increase?
3. increase was	3. The increase was _____.
4. a _____ increase	4. A _____ increase–Wow!
5. that increase	5. That increase is too much for me.
/kwi/	
1. queen of England	1. Who is the queen of England?
2. Queen Elizabeth II	2. Her name is Queen Elizabeth II.
3. Queen Elizabeth I	3. Who was Queen Elizabeth I?
4. queen's grandmother	4. The Queen's grandmother.
5. who's queen.	5. How do you figure out who's queen next?
/gri/	
1. green grass	1. I see a lot of green grass.
2. green trees	2. There're green trees, too.
3. else is green	3. What else is green out there?
4. green eyes	4. Do you have green eyes?
5. green shirt	5. No, but I have a green shirt.
/sli/	
1. to sleep	1. Go to sleep!
2. sleep tight	2. Goodnight, sleep tight.
3. get to sleep	3. I can't get to sleep.
4. lost sleep	4. Lost sleep is hard to find.
5. sleep over	5. Can you sleep over tonight?
/swi/	
1. sweet tooth	1. Do you have a sweet tooth?
2. sweet girl	2. She's really a sweet girl.
3. sugar is sweet	3. Sugar is sweet and _____.
4. sweet and sour	4. I like all candy–sweet and sour.
5. too sweet	5. Some pies are just too sweet.

/i/ CONTEXTS

Distinctive features: high-front, tense, unround
/i/ ***consonant combinations:*** Final position of a stressed syllable

Deep Test

/ri/ real	/ni/ knee	/di/ idea	/mi/ me	/fri/ free
/si/ sea	/gri/ agree	/ʃi/ she	/wi/ we	/θri/ three
/bi/ be	/pi/ people	/hi/ he	/tri/ tree	

Common Words

/ri/	/si/	/bi/	/ni/	/gri/	/pi/	/di/	/ʃi/
real	sea	be	knee	agree	people	idea	she
realize	season	being	neither	degree			
really	see						
reason							

/hi/	/mi/	/wi/	/tri/	/fri/	/θri/
he	me	we	tree	free	three

Everyday Language

Phrases	*Sentences*
/ri/	
1. for real	1. Is that for real?
2. really win	2. Did you really win?
3. reason to go	3. What's the reason to go?
4. I realize	4. I realize that's difficult.
5. really hungry	5. I'm really hungry!
/si/	
1. deep blue sea	1. He sailed the deep blue sea.
2. four seasons	2. There are four seasons.
3. see the way	3. I can see the way now.
4. I see	4. I see what you mean.
5. don't see	5. I don't see why.
/bi/	
1. be good	1. I'll be good.
2. being funny	2. He's being funny.
3. be ready	3. She'll be ready.
4. be there	4. Can you be there?
5. being serious	5. She's being serious.

Phrases	*Sentences*
/ni/	
1. sore knee	1. He's got a sore knee.
2. neither right	2. That's neither right nor wrong.
3. bump your knee	3. Did you bump your knee?
4. bend your knee	4. She can bend her knee.
5. neither one	5. Neither one of those will work.
/gri/	
1. agree with me	1. Don't you agree with me?
2. agree with her	2. I agree with her.
3. all agree	3. We should all agree.
4. doesn't agree	4. She doesn't agree with him.
5. we agree	5. How can we agree to that?
/pi/	
1. many people	1. How many people will be there?
2. full of people	2. The room's full of people.
3. people choose	3. The people choose the president.
4. people like	4. Most people like ice cream.
5. some people	5. Some people don't.
/di/	
1. big idea	1. What's the big idea?
2. whose idea	2. Whose idea was that?
3. which idea	3. Which idea is best?
4. that idea	4. Why pick that idea?
5. your idea	5. Have we heard your idea?
/ʃi/	
1. she did	1. She did it, didn't she?
2. did she	2. What did she do?
3. she do it	3. When did she do it?
4. she could	4. She could have done it today.
5. could she	5. Oh, how could she!
/hi/	
1. he did	1. He did it, didn't he?
2. did he	2. What did he do?
3. he do it	3. When did he do it?
4. he could	4. He could have done it today.
5. could he	5. Oh, how could he?

Phrases	*Sentences*
/mi/	
1. for me	1. He did it for me.
2. gave me	2. They gave me a choice.
3. wants me	3. She wants me to go.
4. needs me	4. He needs me to stay.
5. oh, me	5. Oh, me, oh, my—what to do!
/wi/	
1. we did	1. We did it, didn't we?
2. we certainly did	2. We certainly did it this time.
3. we could	3. We could do it again.
4. will we	4. When will we try?
5. we can	5. Just as soon as we can.
/tri/	
1. pretty tree	1. That's a pretty tree.
2. Christmas tree	2. Let's put up the Christmas tree.
3. apple tree	3. The old apple tree is dead.
4. shade tree	4. Let's find a shade tree.
5. up a tree	5. This thing's got me up a tree!
/fri/	
1. movie is free	1. The movie is free tonight.
2. isn't free	2. The program isn't free, is it?
3. free things	3. Name three free things.
4. are free	4. The best things in life are free!
5. free time	5. Do you have any free time today?
/θri/	
1. three pennies	1. Put three pennies in the meter.
2. three wishes	2. Suppose you had three wishes . . .
3. three times	3. Three times three is _____?
4. three strikes	4. Three strikes and you're out.
5. three-thirty	5. Be ready at three-thirty.

/ɪ/ CONTEXTS

Distinctive features: high-front, lax, unround
/ɪ/ ***consonant combinations:*** Initial position of a stressed syllable

Deep Test

/ɪn/ in	/ɪts/ its	/ɪf/ if	/ɪl/ ill	/ɪntʃ/ inch
/ɪz/ is	/ɪt/ it	/ɪʃ/ issue	/ɪr/ ear	

Common Words

/ɪn/	/ɪz/	/ɪts/	/ɪt/	/ɪf/	/ɪʃ/	/ɪl/	/ɪr/	/ɪntʃ/
in	is	its	it	if	issue	ill	ear	inch
industry								
interest								
into								
within								

Everyday Language

Phrases	*Sentences*
/ɪn/	
1. into the tree	1. He ran into the tree.
2. come in	2. Come in here!
3. interest you	3. Does this interest you?
4. big industry	4. Bubble gum is a big industry.
5. within my power	5. If it's within my power, I will.
/ɪz/	
1. is it	1. Is it ready yet?
2. it isn't	2. No, it isn't.
3. is it almost	3. Is it almost ready?
4. it is	4. Yes, it is.
5. isn't that	5. Isn't that nice!
/ɪts/	
1. it's his	1. It's his book.
2. it's mine	2. No, it's mine.
3. it's not	3. It's not either!
4. it's hers	4. It's hers, I think.
5. it's really not	5. It's really not his.

Phrases	*Sentences*
/ɪt/	
1. is it	1. Is it ready?
2. it isn't	2. No, it isn't.
3. is it almost	3. Is it almost ready?
4. it is	4. Yes, it is.
5. have it	5. May I have it?
/ɪf/	
1. if you can	1. Do it if you can.
2. if you can't	2. If you can't, that's OK.
3. if I fail	3. What happens if I fail?
4. if you fail	4. If you fail, you fail.
5. if you win	5. If you win, you win!
/ɪʃ/	
1. make an issue	1. Don't make an issue of it.
2. first issue	2. Try to get the first issue.
3. issue books	3. Do they issue books?
4. the issue	4. What's the issue?
5. issue a warning	5. Did they issue a warning yet?
/ɪl/	
1. ill feelings	1. No ill feelings, OK?
2. he's ill	2. I think he's ill today.
3. she's ill	3. I hear she's ill, too.
4. you're ill	4. Don't come if you're ill.
5. ill will	5. That's a sign of ill will.
/ɪr/	
1. ear ache	1. I really have an ear ache.
2. eye and ear	2. Who's a good eye and ear doctor?
3. good ear	3. She has a good ear for music.
4. your ear	4. Who said, "Lend me your ear"?
5. earphone	5. You must wear an earphone.
/ɪntʃ/	
1. inch long	1. It's about an inch long.
2. an inch	2. They won't budge an inch.
3. give an inch	3. Give an inch, take a mile!
4. inch along	4. We just try to inch along.
5. over an inch	5. All that fuss over an inch?

/ɪ/ CONTEXTS

Distinctive features: high-front, lax, unround
/ɪ/ ***consonant combinations:*** Initial position of an unstressed syllable

Deep Test

/ɪn/ include /ɪk/ except /ɪt/ itself /ɪg/ example /ɪm/ important

Common Words

/ɪn/	/ɪk/	/ɪt/	/ɪg/	/ɪm/
enjoy	except	itself	example	important
include	expect			
increase	experience			
indeed	explain			
instead	express			

Everyday Language

Phrases	*Sentences*
/ɪn/	
1. enjoy yourself	1. Enjoy yourself, it's later than you think!
2. include taxes	2. That price doesn't include taxes.
3. price increase	3. No, that's just the price increase.
4. other one instead	4. Do you want the other one instead?
5. do indeed	5. I do indeed!
/ɪk/	
1. except that one	1. Everything goes except that one.
2. expect her	2. We expect her anytime now.
3. little experience	3. They have little experience working.
4. explain it	4. Could you explain it again?
5. express yourself	5. Try to express yourself a little better.
/ɪt/	
1. run itself	1. It won't run itself, you know.
2. hurt itself	2. Will it hurt itself?
3. by itself	3. It will get down by itself.
4. clean itself	4. A cat can clean itself without a bath.
5. turn itself	5. Let go and it will turn itself around.

Phrases	*Sentences*
/ɪg/	
1. good example	1. Try to be a good example.
2. bad example	2. How do you tell a bad example?
3. every example	3. Look at every example.
4. each example	4. Can you try each example?
5. one example	5. One example is enough.
/ɪm/	
1. important person	1. Name an important person.
2. important to whom	2. Important to whom—you or me?
3. important to you	3. Important to you, I guess.
4. anyone important	4. I don't know anyone important.
5. you're important	5. You're important—do you know you?

/ɪ/ CONTEXTS

Distinctive features: high-front, lax, unround
/ɪ/ ***consonant combinations:*** Medial position of a stressed syllable

Deep Test

/sɪ/ city	/pɪ/ appear	/θɪ/ thin	/ðɪ/ this	/trɪ/ trip
/bɪ/ big	/tɪ/ until	/brɪ/ bridge	/ʃɪ/ ship	/drɪ/ drink
/fɪ/ fill	/lɪ/ lip	/vɪ/ visit	/tʃɪ/ children	/klɪ/ clear
/wɪ/ will	/kɪ/ kill	/prɪ/ pretty	/nɪ/ near	/kwɪ/ quickly
/mɪ/ admit	/rɪ/ river	/spɪ/ spirit	/hwɪ/ which	/skɪ/ skin
/dɪ/ did	/gɪ/ begin	/stɪ/ stick	/jɪ/ year	/sprɪ/ spring
/hɪ/ hill				

Common Words

/sɪ/	/bɪ/	/fɪ/	/wɪ/	/mɪ/	/dɪ/
city	big	fear	will	admit	condition
consider	bill	fifty	win	middle	dear
sick	bit	figure	wind	milk	did
silver	build	fill	window	million	difference
simple	building	finger	wing	minute	different
since	built	finish	winter	miss	dinner
sing	business	fish	with	permit	distance
single	busy	fit	women		
sister					
sit					
six					
system					

/hɪ/	/pɪ/	/tɪ/	/lɪ/	/kɪ/	/rɪ/	/gɪ/
hear	appear	continue	lift	kill	rich	begin
here	opinion	material	lip	king	ring	give
hill	period	tear	listen	kiss	river	given
him	pick	till	little	kitchen	written	
his	picture	until	live			
history						

/θɪ/	/brɪ/	/vɪ/	/prɪ/	/spɪ/	/stɪ/	/ði/	/ʃɪ/
thin	bridge	village	pretty	experience	stick	this	ship
thing	bring	visit	prince	spirit	still		
think							

/tʃɪ/	/nɪ/	/hwɪ/	/jɪ/	/trɪ/	/drɪ/	/klɪ/	/kwɪ/
children	near	which	year	trip	drink	clear	quickly

/skɪ/	/sprɪ/
skin	spring

Everyday Language

Phrases

/sɪ/

1. big city
2. consider leaving
3. sick today
4. your sister
5. sit by

Sentences

1. I like the big city.
2. Would you consider leaving?
3. I think I'll be sick today.
4. Is your sister named _____?
5. I'd really like to sit by _____.

Phrases	*Sentences*
/bɪ/	
1. pay the bill	1. Someone has to pay the bill.
2. little bit	2. I'd like just a little bit.
3. what building	3. What building do you go to?
4. crazy business	4. This is a crazy business alright.
5. busy day	5. Boy, what a busy day!
/fɪ/	
1. no fear	1. Have no fear, _____ is here!
2. fifty dollars	2. He bet me fifty dollars he could.
3. one finger	3. Hold up one finger.
4. finish first	4. If you finish first, you win.
5. fish story	5. That sounds like a fish story to me.
/wɪ/	
1. I will	1. I will if you will.
2. can't win	2. Some days you just can't win!
3. to the wind	3. Just listen to the wind.
4. with me	4. Why don't you come with me?
5. women are always	5. Women are always _____, aren't they?
/mɪ/	
1. I admit	1. I admit it, you're the best.
2. in the middle	2. You're caught in the middle.
3. million dollars	3. Not for a million dollars!
4. a minute	4. Now just wait a minute.
5. miss you	5. We'll miss you when you're gone.
/dɪ/	
1. one condition	1. She'll do it on one condition.
2. the difference	2. What's the difference?
3. really different	3. Are they really different?
4. from a distance	4. You can't tell from a distance.
5. eat dinner	5. Well, let's eat dinner now.
/hɪ/	
1. hear him	1. I can just hear him tell it.
2. come here	2. Do you think they'll come here?
3. fool him	3. You won't fool him with that.
4. his tricks	4. She's up to his tricks.
5. ancient history	5. First grade seems like ancient history.

Phrases	*Sentences*
/pɪ/	
1. appear foolish	1. We don't want to appear foolish.
2. your opinion	2. That's just your opinion.
3. fourth period	3. We can do it fourth period today.
4. pick a time	4. Let's pick a time now.
5. pretty picture	5. They make a pretty picture together.
/tɪ/	
1. continue this	1. Continue this tomorrow.
2. new material	2. New material is hard to work with.
3. tear it	3. You'll tear it if you pull.
4. until five	4. We don't close until five.
5. 'til tomorrow	5. Wait 'til tomorrow, then try it.
/lɪ/	
1. lift your spirits	1. The news will lift your spirits!
2. button your lip	2. What does "button your lip" mean?
3. listen carefully	3. Listen carefully, then you'll know.
4. little bit	4. Move it just a little bit.
5. live a little	5. Let's live a little!
/kɪ/	
1. kill me	1. My dad'll kill me if he finds out.
2. who's king	2. If there's a queen bee, who's king?
3. a little kiss	3. Give me a little kiss.
4. in the kitchen	4. It's hot in the kitchen.
5. kill you	5. Go ahead, it won't kill you!
/rɪ/	
1. be rich	1. I'd like to be rich.
2. class ring	2. Did you get your class ring?
3. longest river	3. What's the longest river?
4. written her	4. Have you written her yet?
5. really rich	5. That pie is really rich!
/gɪ/	
1. we begin	1. Today we begin a new unit.
2. give me	2. Give me time; I'm hurrying.
3. given you	3. They've given you plenty already.
4. begin again	4. Then I'll have to begin again.
5. to begin	5. You have ten minutes to begin working.

Phrases	*Sentences*
/θɪ/	
1. so thin	1. She looks so thin!
2. a thing	2. She doesn't eat a thing.
3. I think	3. I think she should stop dieting.
4. too thin	4. You can be too thin.
5. think so	5. I think so, too.
/brɪ/	
1. bridge the gap	1. We'll try to bridge the gap.
2. bring me	2. Bring me the evidence.
3. bring it	3. Bring it when you come tonight.
4. longest bridge	4. What's the longest bridge?
5. tallest bridge	5. What's the tallest bridge?
/vɪ/	
1. small village	1. It's just a small village.
2. like a visit	2. I'd like to visit it anyway.
3. second village	3. It's the second village.
4. visit often	4. Do you visit often?
5. first visit	5. No, this is my first visit.
/prɪ/	
1. as pretty as	1. She's as pretty as a _____.
2. a prince	2. He's a prince of a fellow!
3. about a prince	3. Do you know a story about a prince?
4. pretty moon	4. What a pretty moon!
5. pretty soon	5. They better come pretty soon.
/spɪ/	
1. years of experience	1. It takes years of experience.
2. spirit is willing	2. The spirit is willing but _____.
3. good experience	3. You can't beat good experience.
4. scary experience	4. What a scary experience!
5. school spirit	5. What happened to our school spirit?
/stɪ/	
1. stick to it	1. Stick to it and you'll finish.
2. still working	2. I'm still working on the first problem.
3. big stick	3. Who said "Carry a big stick"?
4. still as glass	4. The lake is still as glass.
5. still time	5. There's still time to go.

Phrases	*Sentences*
/ði/	
1. this and that	1. We talked about this and that.
2. this time	2. This time we get it right!
3. this place	3. This place is getting to me.
4. this way	4. Go this way this time.
5. this is	5. This is the one, alright.
/ʃɪ/	
1. ship out	1. Shape up or ship out!
2. the ship	2. Who said "Don't give up the ship"?
3. ship shape	3. Everything is ship shape.
4. ship it	4. They won't ship it for two weeks.
5. biggest ship	5. What's the biggest ship?
/tʃɪ/	
1. like children	1. Sometimes they act like children.
2. children should	2. Children should be seen and _____.
3. for children	3. Christmas is for children.
4. children go	4. Let the children go first.
5. two children	5. They have two children–a boy and girl.
/nɪ/	
1. is near	1. Your time is near.
2. near here	2. Do you live near here?
3. nearby	3. My house is nearby.
4. near the ocean	4. I'd like to live near the ocean.
5. getting near	5. We're getting near the place.
/hwɪ/	
1. which way	1. Which way should we go?
2. which is	2. Which is best?
3. which one	3. Which one did you choose?
4. which kind	4. It doesn't matter which kind.
5. which color	5. Which color matches your coat?
/jɪ/	
1. year has	1. The year has just started.
2. long year	2. Think it will be a long year?
3. last year	3. Last year seemed short.
4. every year	4. Time goes faster every year.
5. new year	5. Happy New Year!

Phrases	*Sentences*
/trɪ/	
1. plan a trip	1. Did you plan a trip?
2. long trip	2. Will it be a long trip?
3. short trip	3. Just time for a short trip.
4. one trip	4. One trip is not enough.
5. second trip	5. Plan your second trip now.
/drɪ/	
1. get a drink	1. Where can we get a drink of water?
2. drink a lot	2. I drink a lot of milk.
3. drink coffee	3. Do you drink coffee?
4. I drink	4. I drink about _____ cups a day.
5. soft drink	5. _____ is a kind of soft drink.
/klɪ/	
1. clear to me	1. Can you make it clear to me?
2. clear up	2. Maybe the weather will clear up.
3. clear the room	3. Clear the room and let's dance.
4. clear the way	4. Here they come—clear the way!
5. clear day	5. Tomorrow will be a clear day.
/kwɪ/	
1. how quickly	1. See how quickly you can do it.
2. work quickly	2. Try to work quickly.
3. do it quickly	3. There's no way to do it quickly.
4. runs quickly	4. He runs quickly enough to win.
5. go quickly	5. Go quickly and see.
/skɪ/	
1. pretty skin	1. She has pretty skin.
2. skin of his teeth	2. He made it by the skin of his teeth.
3. skin you	3. He'll skin you alive!
4. dry skin	4. What's good for dry skin?
5. onion skin	5. It's as thin as onion skin.
/sprɪ/	
1. spring has	1. Spring has sprung!
2. until spring	2. I can't wait until spring.
3. broken spring	3. It has a broken spring.
4. wind the spring	4. Can you wind the spring?
5. new spring	5. Put in a new spring.

/ɪ/ CONTEXTS

Distinctive features: high-front, lax, unround
/ɪ/ ***consonant combinations:*** Medial position of an unstressed syllable

Deep Test

/tɪ/ native	/nɪ/ business	/kɪ/ market	/zɪ/ music	/dʒɪ/ subject
/θɪ/ anything	/wɪ/ within	/vɪ/ service	/hɪ/ himself	/lɪ/ public

Common Words

/tɪ/	/θɪ/	/nɪ/	/wɪ/	/kɪ/	/vɪ/
captain	anything	business	always	market	service
native	everything	evening	within		
notice	something	morning	without		
practice					

/zɪ/	/hɪ/	/dʒɪ/	/lɪ/
music	himself	subject	public

Everyday Language

Phrases	*Sentences*
/tɪ/	
1. team captain	1. Who's the team captain?
2. read the notice	2. Did you read the notice?
3. practice tonight	3. We have band practice tonight.
4. practice makes perfect	4. As they say, "Practice makes perfect."
5. native crafts	5. They sell native crafts here.
/θɪ/	
1. anything goes	1. Some days anything goes.
2. everything goes	2. Some days everything goes wrong.
3. something goes	3. Let's hope something goes right.
4. for anything.	4. I'll hope for anything!
5. everything will	5. Everything will come out just right.
/nɪ/	
1. monkey business	1. Remember–no monkey business.
2. this evening	2. Lets do the report this evening.
3. until morning	3. I'd rather wait until morning.
4. your business	4. Well, it's none of your business.
5. my business	5. I'll make it my business.

Phrases	*Sentences*
/wɪ/	
1. always wanted	1. I always wanted a red coat.
2. do without	2. You can do without it this time.
3. without it	3. I did without it last year.
4. from within	4. The feelings must come from within.
5. within my power	5. If it's within my power, I will.
/kɪ/	
1. stock market	1. Do you play that stock market?
2. market work	2. How does the market work?
3. market goes up	3. Sometimes the market goes up.
4. market goes down	4. Sometimes the market goes down.
5. market is risky	5. Playing the market is risky.
/vɪ/	
1. good service	1. They have good service here.
2. service station	2. I like this service station.
3. bad service	3. Sometimes you get bad service.
4. friendly service	4. I don't mind if it's friendly service.
5. any service	5. Any service is better than no service.
/zɪ/	
1. good music	1. You can't beat good music.
2. kinds of music	2. I like all kinds of music.
3. music major	3. I wish I were a music major.
4. music to my ears	4. Those words are music to my ears.
5. sweet music	5. That's sweet music!
/hɪ/	
1. go himself	1. He'll have to go himself.
2. for himself	2. He'll keep one for himself.
3. do it himself	3. He must do it himself.
4. see himself	4. He can see himself in the mirror.
5. one for himself	5. It's one for himself and one for you.
/dʒɪ/	
1. touchy subject	1. That's a touchy subject.
2. one subject	2. I'm taking only one subject.
3. the subject	3. The subject for today is dogs.
4. my subject	4. Ladies and gentlemen, my subject is you.
5. another subject	5. Let's turn to another subject now.

Phrases	*Sentences*
/lɪ/	
1. public eye	1. She's in the public eye.
2. make it public	2. When will they make it public?
3. public knowledge	3. It isn't really public knowledge.
4. John Q. Public	4. Who is "John Q. Public"?
5. public nuisance	5. Trash is a public nuisance.

/ɪ/ CONTEXTS

Distinctive features: high-front, lax, unround
/ɪ/ ***consonant combinations:*** Final position of an unstressed syllable

Deep Test

/rɪ/ every	/lɪ/ only	/mɪ/ army	/prɪ/ prepare
/bɪ/ baby	/tɪ/ party	/nɪ/ company	/blɪ/ probably
/dɪ/ demand	/trɪ/ country		

Common Words

/rɪ/	/bɪ/	/dɪ/	/lɪ/	/tɪ/	/trɪ/
century	baby	decide	certainly	article	country
every	because	declare	daily	beauty	industry
everything	became	degree	early	duty	
history	become	demand	especially	fifty	
receive	before	department	family	party	
refuse	began	desire	nearly	society	
regard	begin	destroy	only	thirty	
remain	behind	Indian	quickly	twenty	
remember	beside	lady	suddenly		
remove	beyond				
reply					
report					
require					
result					
return					
story					

/mɪ/	/nɪ/	/prɪ/	/blɪ/
army	company	prepare	probably
enemy			

Phrases	*Sentences*
/rɪ/	
1. every day	1. Every day in every way, we do better.
2. everything well	2. She does everything well.
3. history class	3. Where do you sit in history class?
4. remember it	4. Try to remember it this time.
5. story about	5. What's the story about?
/bɪ/	
1. baby him	1. Let's not baby him.
2. because he's	2. Because he's a big boy now.
3. did before	3. We always did before now.
4. to begin	4. It's a good time to begin.
5. beside myself	5. I'm just beside myself!
/dɪ/	
1. could decide	1. I wish I could decide.
2. much demand	2. There isn't much demand.
3. which department	3. Which department handles this?
4. destroy me	4. His jokes destroy me!
5. real lady	5. She's a real lady.
/lɪ/	
1. early to bed	1. Early to bed and _____.
2. especially nice	2. It's especially nice this year.
3. daily dozen	3. Did you do your daily dozen?
4. certainly did	4. I most certainly did!
5. only one	5. Just think–only one more week!
/tɪ/	
1. raving beauty	1. She's no raving beauty, you know.
2. your duty	2. If it's your duty, then do it.
3. fifty dollars	3. I bet you fifty dollars I can.
4. a party	4. Can you come to a party tonight?
5. twenty years old	5. He's about twenty years old.
/trɪ/	
1. free country	1. It's a free country.
2. in the country	2. I'd like to live in the country.
3. from the industry	3. Me, too–away from the industry.
4. country kitchen	4. I want a house with a country kitchen.
5. country living	5. Country living sounds great!

Phrases	*Sentences*
/mɪ/	
1. joined the army	1. Did you know that _____ joined the army?
2. flight the enemy	2. Going to fight the enemy, huh?
3. this army	3. Not in this army.
4. which army	4. Which army did he join?
5. Salvation Army	5. The Salvation Army!
/nɪ/	
1. had company	1. We had company this weekend.
2. nice company	2. Nice company, would you say?
3. good company	3. I'd call them good company.
4. much company	4. We don't have much company.
5. company comes	5. Company comes at odd times.
/prɪ/	
1. to prepare	1. Time to prepare lunch.
2. easy to prepare	2. Let's have eggs; they're easy to prepare.
3. I'll prepare	3. I'll prepare enough for three.
4. wouldn't prepare	4. I wouldn't prepare that much.
5. bother to prepare	5. Why bother to prepare any at all?
/blɪ/	
1. probably right	1. You're probably right.
2. probably wrong	2. I'm probably wrong.
3. not probably	3. Possibly but not probably.
4. probably tell	4. They'll probably tell us today.
5. probably hear	5. No, we'll probably hear tomorrow.

/e/ CONTEXTS

Distinctive features: high-mid-front, tense, unround
/e/ ***consonant combinations:*** Initial position of a stressed syllable

Deep Test

/e/ able   /et/ eight   /edʒ/ age

Common Words

/e/	/et/	/edʒ/
able	eight	age

Everyday Language

Phrases	*Sentences*
/e/	
1. ready and able	1. He's ready and able to work.
2. be able	2. Will you be able to go?
3. we're able	3. We're able to do better.
4. able-bodied man	4. He's an able-bodied man.
5. able to see	5. We'll be able to see from here.
/et/	
1. half past eight	1. Half past eight–don't be late!
2. eight hours	2. It's an eight hour a day job.
3. eight days	3. Sometimes I need eight days in a week.
4. eight times eight	4. Eight times eight is _____.
5. eight ways	5. There are eight ways to swim–name two.
/edʒ/	
1. what age	1. At what age did you start school?
2. must age	2. Cheese must age to be good.
3. age four	3. He started playing at age four.
4. Golden Age	4. What was the "Golden Age"?
5. show her age	5. She doesn't show her age.

/e/ CONTEXTS

Distinctive features: high-mid-front, tense, unround
/e/ ***consonant combinations:*** Medial position of a stressed syllable

Deep Test

/te/ contain	/we/ wave	/fe/ face	/stre/ straight	/kle/ claim
/re/ race	/ke/ came	/ʃe/ shade	/be/ base	/gre/ great
/pe/ paid	/me/ made	/ple/ place	/tʃe/ change	/fre/ afraid
/ge/ game	/le/ lake	/tre/ trade	/ne/ name	/spe/ space
/se/ safe	/de/ date	/ste/ state	/bre/ break	/ske/ escape

Common Words

/te/	/re/	/pe/	/ge/	/se/	/we/	/ke/
contain	race	page	gain	safe	wait	came
obtain	railroad	paid	game	sail	waste	became
take	rain	pain	gate	same	wave	case
taken	raise	paint	gave	save	weight	
taste	rate					

/me/	/le/	/de/	/fe/	/ʃe/	/ple/	/tre/	/stre/
made	laid	danger	face	shade	place	trade	straight
make	lake	date	fail	shape	plain	train	strange
remain	late						

/ste/	/be/	/tʃe/	/ne/	/bre/	/kle/	/gre/	/fre/
state	base	change	name	break	claim	great	afraid

/spe/	/ske/
space	escape

Everyday Language

Phrases	*Sentences*
/te/	
1. take a walk	1. Let's take a walk.
2. taken your medicine	2. Have you taken your medicine?
3. like the taste	3. I like the taste!
4. contain sugar	4. Does it contain sugar?
5. take a break	5. Time to take a break.
/re/	
1. wild race	1. That was a wild race!
2. near the railroad	2. They live near the railroad.
3. rain today	3. Oh, it *would* rain today!
4. raise the money	4. How will we raise the money?
5. lower rate	5. Let's ask for a lower rate.
/pe/	
1. page ten	1. Turn to page ten.
2. paid my way	2. I paid my way to the game.
3. any pain	3. Do you have any pain?
4. paint it	4. I'd paint it yellow.
5. last page	5. This is the last page–thank goodness!

Phrases	*Sentences*
/ge/	
1. one yard gain	1. That was a one yard gain.
2. some game	2. This is really some game!
3. big gate	3. A big crowd means a big gate.
4. gave it away	4. They just gave it away.
5. next game	5. Just wait 'til the next game.
/se/	
1. like to sail	1. Do you like to sail?
2. is it safe	2. Is it safe to sail alone?
3. same as	3. Same as swimming–better with two.
4. save me	4. Could you save me from drowning?
5. you're safe	5. You're safe with me.
/we/	
1. wait to go	1. I just can't wait to go.
2. waste time	2. Don't waste time.
3. wave as	3. Wave as you go by.
4. lose weight	4. Did you lose weight last week?
5. wait for	5. Wait for me, I'm coming!
/ke/	
1. became of	1. What became of George?
2. came late	2. He came late.
3. difficult case	3. He's a difficult case.
4. came last	4. We came last year.
5. whole case	5. Can you buy a whole case?
/me/	
1. made it clear	1. I thought we made it clear.
2. make it clearer	2. Try to make it clearer.
3. two remain	3. One goes and two remain.
4. got it made	4. Boy, you've got it made!
5. make it	5. We can make it now.
/le/	
1. laid an egg	1. The show laid an egg!
2. go the lake	2. Let's go to the lake.
3. late again	3. Well, she's late again.
4. laid it down	4. I laid it down here.
5. late show	5. Want to see the late show?

Phrases	*Sentences*
/de/	
1. no danger	1. There's no danger of that.
2. have a date	2. Do you have a date?
3. date today	3. What's the date today?
4. make a date	4. Let's make a date.
5. danger sign	5. See the danger sign?
/fe/	
1. dirty face	1. What a dirty face!
2. face her	2. I can't face her.
3. fail now	3. You can't fail now.
4. face up	4. Face up to it!
5. don't fail	5. Don't fail me!
/ʃe/	
1. pull the shade	1. Pull the shade, please.
2. shape up	2. Shape up or _____.
3. a shape	3. What a shape!
4. shade small	4. It's just a shade small.
5. he'll shape	5. Maybe he'll shape up.
/ple/	
1. nice place	1. This is a nice place.
2. plain or	2. Plain or fancy—I like it.
3. what place	3. What place did you say?
4. plain vanilla	4. I like plain vanilla.
5. place to sleep	5. He just needs a place to sleep.
/tre/	
1. trade you	1. I'll trade you.
2. next train	2. When's the next train?
3. trade cars	3. He's going to trade cars.
4. train him	4. Train him to sit up.
5. poor trade	5. It's a poor trade.
/ste/	
1. sorry state	1. What a sorry state!
2. biggest state	2. The biggest state is _____.
3. smallest state	3. The smallest state is _____.
4. warmest state	4. The warmest state is _____.
5. best state	5. The best state is _____.

Phrases	*Sentences*
/stre/	
1. straight down	1. Go straight down and turn left.
2. strange things	2. Strange things are happening!
3. strange places	3. Strange places are scary.
4. be straight	4. It has to be straight.
5. straight and narrow	5. Walk the straight and narrow!
/be/	
1. first base	1. He won't get to first base.
2. base that	2. What do you base that on?
3. base it	3. I base it on fact.
4. second base	4. He stole second base.
4. the base	5. We broke the base.
/tʃe/	
1. have to change	1. You'll have to change.
2. can't change	2. I can't change.
3. could change	3. You could change.
4. won't change	4. I won't change.
5. only change	5. Only change will make it better.
/ne/	
1. your name	1. What's your name?
2. first name	2. My first name?
3. last name	3. Yes, and last name.
4. middle name	4. I have no middle name.
5. third name	5. Who needs a third name?
/bre/	
1. a break	1. Give me a break.
2. deserve a break	2. Do you deserve a break?
3. little break	3. Everyone needs a little break.
4. kind of break	4. What kind of break?
5. coffee break	5. A coffee break!
/kle/	
1. claim to fame	1. What's your claim to fame?
2. don't claim	2. I don't claim to be famous.
3. must claim	3. You must claim something.
4. claim to be	4. I claim to be honest.
5. worth a claim	5. That's worth a claim.

Phrases	*Sentences*
/gre/	
1. look great	1. You look great!
2. feel great	2. I feel great!
3. makes you great	3. What makes you great?
4. great help	4. You're a great help!
5. great big	5. That's a great big lie!
/fre/	
1. afraid of	1. Are you afraid of snakes?
2. mostly afraid	2. I'm mostly afraid of ____.
3. be afraid	3. It's good to be afraid sometimes.
4. always afraid	4. Are you always afraid?
5. I'm afraid	5. I'm afraid so!
/spe/	
1. outer space	1. Outer space is weird!
2. understand outer space	2. I don't understand outer space.
3. like outer space	3. It looks like outer space.
4. in outer space	4. Are we in outer space, too?
5. be outer space	5. It must be outer space.
/ske/	
1. can't escape	1. You can't escape work.
2. try to escape	2. Some people try to escape.
3. let's escape	3. Let's escape to an island.
4. we escape	4. How can we escape?
5. escape hatch	5. Go through the escape hatch.

/e/ CONTEXTS

Distinctive features: high-mid-front, tense, unround
/e/ ***consonant combinations:*** Final position of a stressed syllable

Deep Test

/ne/ nation	/be/ bay	/we/ way	/ðe/ they	/ple/ play
/le/ lay	/de/ day	/ste/ stay	/se/ say	/gre/ gray
/pe/ pay	/fe/ famous	/te/ table	/me/ may	

Common Words

/ne/	/le/	/pe/	/be/	/de/	/fe/	/we/
nation	lay	paper	baby	day	famous	away
native	labor	pay	bay	today	favor	way
nature	lady					
neighbor						

/ste/	/te/	/ðe/	/se/	/me/	/ple/	/gre/
station	table	they	say	may	play	gray
stay						

Everyday Language

Phrases	*Sentences*
/ne/	
1. one nation	1. "One nation, under God."
2. native dance	2. Can you do a native dance?
3. with nature	3. Let's commune with nature!
4. my neighbor	4. He's my neighbor.
5. good neighbor	5. Be a good neighbor.
/le/	
1. lay me	1. Now I lay me down to sleep.
2. hard labor	2. Hard labor pays off.
3. nice lady	3. She's a nice lady.
4. lay your books	4. Don't lay your books there.
5. labor of love	5. It's a labor of love.
/pe/	
1. seen the paper	1. Have you seen the paper?
2. today's paper	2. Do you mean today's paper?
3. morning paper	3. Yes, I mean the morning paper.
4. evening paper	4. Here's the evening paper.
5. that paper	5. I've seen that paper.
/be/	
1. new baby	1. They have a new baby.
2. baby boy	2. It's a baby boy.
3. baby girl	3. We have a baby girl.
4. good baby	4. A good baby is fun.
5. any baby	5. Any baby is a good baby.

Phrases	*Sentences*
/de/	
1. today is	1. Today is a good time to start.
2. day time	2. Day time is best.
3. what day	3. What day will you come?
4. today or tomorrow	4. Today or tomorrow, I'm not sure.
5. come today	5. Try to come today.
/fe/	
1. famous people	1. Famous people are friendly.
2. a favor	2. Do me a favor?
3. famous place	3. This is a famous place.
4. famous person	4. The most famous person I know is _____.
5. him a favor	5. Do him a favor and help.
/we/	
1. get away	1. Get away from me!
2. long way	2. It's a long way.
3. which way	3. Which way from here?
4. going away	4. Hurray, I'm going away!
5. long way away	5. Are you going a long way away?
/ste/	
1. stay awhile	1. Please stay awhile.
2. long stay	2. We're in for a long stay.
3. station is	3. The station is closed.
4. service station	4. The service station should fix it.
5. stay open	5. Do they stay open late?
/te/	
1. on the table	1. Lay your cards on the table.
2. set the table	2. Please set the table.
3. under the table	3. It's under the table.
4. in the table	4. Look in the table drawer.
5. table and chairs	5. We need a table and chairs.
/ðe/	
1. they say	1. They say they can't.
2. they won't	2. I bet they won't.
3. they could	3. I know they could.
4. they will	4. Maybe they will.
5. they'd better	5. By golly, they'd better!

Phrases	*Sentences*
/se/	
1. did he say	1. What did he say?
2. say anything	2. He didn't say anything.
3. say something	3. Why won't he say something?
4. can't say	4. I can't say.
5. say it	5. I'd say it to his face.
/me/	
1. may go	1. I may go later.
2. may I	2. May I tell her?
3. may know	3. He may know how.
4. may happen	4. It may happen.
5. may rain	5. It may rain today.
/ple/	
1. play around	1. Don't play around.
2. child's play	2. This is child's play.
3. playground	3. Where's the playground?
4. the play	4. The play is tonight.
5. no play	5. All work and no play . . .
/gre/	
1. gray day	1. It's a gray day.
2. gray coat	2. Where's my gray coat?
3. pretty gray	3. Her hair is pretty gray.
4. gray cars	4. Gray cars look expensive.
5. kind of gray	5. It turned kind of gray.

/ɛ/ CONTEXTS

Distinctive features: low-mid-front, lax, unround
/ɛ/ ***consonant combinations:*** Initial position of a stressed syllable

Deep Test

/ɛv/ ever	/ɛ/ effort	/ɛdʒ/ edge	/ɛnd/ end	/ɛls/ else
/ɛn/ any	/ɛg/ egg	/ɛr/ air		

Common Words

/ɛv/	/ɛn/	/ɛ/	/ɛg/	/ɛdʒ/	/ɛr/	/ɛnd/	/ɛls/
ever	any	effort	egg	edge	air	end	else
every	anything						
everything	enemy						
however	enter						
whatever							

Everyday Language

Phrases	*Sentences*
/ɛv/	
1. ever see	1. Will I ever see him?
2. every day	2. Probably every day.
3. has everything	3. He has everything.
4. whatever you say	4. Whatever you say, I'll do.
5. when however	5. Don't ask me when, however.
/ɛn/	
1. have any	1. We don't have any.
2. anything goes	2. Anything goes here.
3. an enemy	3. I haven't an enemy in the world!
4. don't enter	4. There's a "Don't Enter" sign on it.
5. mean anything	5. That doesn't mean anything.
/ɛ/	
1. the effort	1. It's not worth the effort.
2. much effort	2. How much effort?
3. our effort	3. All our effort.
4. lot of effort	4. That's a lot of effort.
5. has the effort	5. Who has the effort?
/ɛg/	
1. an egg	1. I'd like an egg.
2. want the egg	2. How do you want the egg?
3. my egg	3. I have my egg _____.
4. one egg	4. One egg, comin' up!
5. egg a day	5. I have an egg a day.
/ɛdʒ/	
1. the edge	1. We have the edge on this.
2. near the edge	2. Don't get near the edge.
3. thin edge	3. It's a thin edge.
4. edge may	4. The edge may break.
5. around the edge	5. Go around the edge.

Phrases	*Sentences*
/ɛr/	
1. thin air	1. It's like thin air.
2. air is cool	2. The air is cool.
3. some air	3. Give me some air.
4. the air	4. He gave me the air.
5. air out	5. Let's air out this place!
/ɛnd/	
1. living end	1. She's the living end!
2. near the end	2. We're near the end.
3. does it end	3. How does it end?
4. end is	4. The end is coming.
5. end soon	5. I hope it will end soon.
/ɛls/	
1. someone else	1. Ask someone else.
2. no one else	2. There's no one else to ask.
3. what else	3. What else can we do?
4. somewhere else	4. We can go somewhere else.
5. where else	5. Where else is there?

/ɛ/ CONTEXTS

Distinctive features: low-mid-front, lax, unround
/ɛ/ ***consonant combinations:*** Medial position of a stressed syllable

Deep Test

/sɛ/ set	/fɛ/ fell	/dɛ/ dead	/vɛ/ very	/klɛ/ declare
/mɛ/ met	/ðɛ/ then	/hwɛ/ when	/tʃɛ/ chair	/kwɛ/ question
/lɛ/ led	/dʒɛ/ object	/jɛ/ yes	/twɛ/ twelve	/sprɛ/ spread
/hɛ/ head	/wɛ/ well	/prɛ/ press	/stɛ/ step	/strɛ/ strength
/rɛ/ red	/tɛ/ tell	/frɛ/ fresh	/plɛ/ pleasant	/skwɛ/ square
/gɛ/ get	/nɛ/ neck	/pɛ/ paid	/ʃɛ/ share	
/bɛ/ bed	/spɛ/ spend	/kɛ/ care	/drɛ/ dress	

Common Words

/sɛ/	/mɛ/	/lɛ/	/hɛ/	/rɛ/	/gɛ/
accept	many	led	hair	already	again
cent	measure	left	head	direct	against
center	member	leg	health	direction	forget
century	men	length	heaven	ready	get
except	mention	less	heavy	record	guess
herself	met	let	held	red	together
himself	method	letter	help	rest	
itself	remember	unless			
myself					
said					
second					
sell					
send					
sense					
sent					
set					
settle					
seven					
several					
success					
yourself					

/bɛ/	/fɛ/	/ðɛ/	/dʒɛ/	/wɛ/	/tɛ/
bear	affair	their	general	wear	attempt
bed	fair	them	gentle	weather	attention
been	fell	themselves	gentlemen	well	tell
best	fellow	then	object	went	ten
better	felt	there	suggest	west	

/nɛ/	/spɛ/	/dɛ/	/hwɛ/	/jɛ/	/prɛ/
necessary	especially	dare	when	yellow	present
neck	expect	dead	where	yes	president
never	special	death	whether	yet	press
next	spend				

/frɛ/	/pɛ/	/kɛ/	/vɛ/	/tʃɛ/	/twɛ/	/stɛ/
fresh	pair	care	various	chair	twelve	instead
friend	prepare	kept	very	check	twenty	step

/plɛ/	/ʃɛ/	/drɛ/	/klɛ/	/kwɛ/	/sprɛ/	/strɛ/	/skwɛ/
pleasant	share	dress	declare	question	spread	strength	square
pleasure							

Everyday Language

Phrases	*Sentences*
/sɛ/	
1. have a cent	1. I don't have a cent.
2. in the center	2. Put it in the center.
3. I said	3. I said I would.
4. sent a card	4. We sent a card.
5. several ways	5. You can go several ways.
/mɛ/	
1. many people	1. Do you know many people?
2. be a member	2. You can be a member.
3. members only	3. Members only—OK?
4. we met	4. We met last year.
5. men only	5. The sign says "Men Only."
/lɛ/	
1. shake a leg	1. Shake a leg—we're late.
2. let me	2. Let me help you.
3. turn left	3. Turn left in two blocks.
4. a letter	4. A letter should do it.
4. new length	5. It's the new length.
/hɛ/	
1. your hair	1. Who does your hair?
2. heaven help	2. Heaven help us!
3. held up	3. Did you get held up?
4, needs help	4. She needs help.
5. head start	5. We got a head start.
/rɛ/	
1. rest room	1. Where's the rest room?
2. I'm ready	2. I'm ready when you are.
3. for the record	3. Just for the record, No.
4. red light	4. Watch for the red light.
5. need a rest	5. We need a rest.
/gɛ/	
1. not again	1. Oh, no, not again!
2. against me	2. Don't hold it against me.
3. forget it	3. Forget it, I'll go.
4. guess so	4. I guess so.
5. came together	5. They came together.

Phrases	*Sentences*
/bɛ/	
1. in bed	1. She's in bed now.
2. been gone	2. I've been gone two days.
3. best suit	3. Wear your best suit.
4. better be	4. It had better be good.
5. bear it	5. Grin and bear it.
/fɛ/	
1. fair weather	1. Fair weather today, they say.
2. felt better	2. I never felt better.
3. fair fight	3. It was a fair fight.
4. that fellow	4. That fellow is first.
5. slipped and fell	5. He slipped and fell on the ice.
/ðɛ/	
1. let them	1. Let them go.
2. do it themselves	2. They can do it themselves.
3. then rest	3. Work, then rest.
4. there you	4. There you are!
5. their time	5. Their time is up.
/dʒɛ/	
1. gentle person	1. He's a gentle person.
2. gentlemen be	2. Gentlemen—be seated!
3. don't object	3. I don't object.
4. they suggest	4. They suggest we fly.
5. general rule	5. It's the general rule.
/wɛ/	
1. should I wear	1. What should I wear?
2. bad weather	2. It's bad weather.
3. wear something	3. Well, wear something warm.
4. go west	4. Let's go west where it's warm.
5. wear a	5. Then I can wear a bikini!
/tɛ/	
1. wants attention	1. He just wants attention.
2. tell him	2. Don't tell him now.
3. ten after	3. It's only ten after.
4. no attempt	4. She made no attempt.
5. attention please	5. May we have your attention, please?

Phrases	*Sentences*
/nɛ/	
1. necessary evil	1. It's a necessary evil.
2. neck out	2. You can stick your neck out.
3. never will	3. I never will!
4. next time	4. Maybe.I'll go next time.
5. said never	5. No, I said *never*!
/spɛ/	
1. don't expect	1. Don't expect miracles!
2. special tool	2. It takes a special tool.
3. spend money	3. We spend money like water!
4. especially nice	4. It's especially nice now.
5. expect trouble	5. Do you expect trouble?
/dɛ/	
1. wouldn't dare	1. You wouldn't dare!
2. dead duck	2. He's a dead duck.
3. death of me	3. She'll be the death of me.
4. dare you	4. I dare you!
5. slow death	5. That would be a slow death.
/hwɛ/	
1. when should	1. When should we go?
2. where should	2. Where should we go?
3. whether you want	3. Go whether you want to or not.
4. when I want	4. I will when I want to.
5. where did	5. Where did you put it?
/jɛ/	
1. yellow seems	1. Yellow seems happy.
2. yes I know	2. Yes, I know that.
3. have it yet	3. We can't have it yet.
4. yellow one	4. Take the yellow one.
5. yes or no	5. Well, yes or no?
/prɛ/	
1. present conditions	1. Present conditions won't let us.
2. who's president	2. Who's president of the class?
3. press your luck	3. Don't press your luck.
4. small present	4. Just a small present will do.
5. be president	5. I'd like to be president.

Phrases	*Sentences*
/frɛ/	
1. fresh food	1. This is fresh food.
2. your friend	2. Is he your friend?
3. friend of mine	3. He's no friend of mine.
4. fresh start	4. Let's make a fresh start.
5. friend or	5. Are you friend or foe?
/pɛ/	
1. to prepare	1. It's hard to prepare.
2. one pair	2. One pair should do.
3. buy a pair	3. You have to buy a pair.
4. prepare it	4. He'll prepare it for us.
5. this pair	5. This pair is expensive.
/kɛ/	
1. don't care	1. I don't care.
2. should care	2. You should care.
3. he kept	3. He kept his promise.
4. could care	4. He could care less.
5. kept mine	5. I kept mine, too.
/vɛ/	
1. very sorry	1. I'm very sorry.
2. various ways	2. There are various ways.
3. very often	3. We don't very often.
4. very much	4. Thank you very much.
5. various people	5. Various people know.
/tʃɛ/	
1. a chair	1. Have a chair!
2. check it out	2. Better check it out.
3. check with	3. Check with me first.
4. another chair	4. We need another chair.
5. take a chair	5. Will you take a check?
/twɛ/	
1. twelve times	1. Twelve times twelve is _____.
2. twenty dollars	2. Twenty dollars is a lot.
3. twelve noon	3. It's twelve noon.
4. twenty people	4. Twenty people can go.
5. twenty plus	5. Twenty plus twelve is _____.

Phrases	*Sentences*
/stɛ/	
1. instead of	1. Instead of loafing–work!
2. step right	2. Step right up!
3. me instead	3. Take me instead!
4. first step	4. This is the first step.
5. step backward	5. It's a giant step backward.
/plɛ/	
1. pleasant enough	1. He's pleasant enough.
2. pleasant dreams	2. Pleasant dreams, everyone!
3. a pleasure	3. It'd be a pleasure.
4. pleasant trip	4. Have a pleasant trip.
5. with pleasure	5. I will, with pleasure!
/ʃɛ/	
1. my share	1. What's my share?
2. fair share	2. Is it a fair share?
3. whose share	3. Whose share is this?
4. I'll share	4. I'll share mine.
5. won't share	5. They won't share it.
/drɛ/	
1. new dress	1. Is that a new dress?
2. dress well	2. You dress well.
3. dress up	3. Do we have to dress up?
4. dress quickly	4. You'll have to dress quickly.
5. dress now	5. We'd better dress now.
/klɛ/	
1. declare war	1. They may declare war.
2. declare it	2. Declare it finished!
3. declare you	3. I declare you king!
4. hereby declare	4. We hereby declare you a member.
5. I declare	5. I declare, you've changed!
/kwɛ/	
1. no question	1. There's no question about it.
2. I question	2. I question that.
3. the question	3. What's the question?
4. which question	4. Which question did you miss?
5. that question	5. That question was hard.

Phrases	*Sentences*
/sprɛ/	
1. we're spread	1. We're spread too thin.
2. spread it	2. Spread it on thick!
3. spread out	3. Let's spread out and look.
4. bedspread	4. You need a new bedspread.
5. spread your wings	5. Spread your wings and fly!
/strɛ/	
1. need strength	1. You'll need strength.
2. takes strength	2. It takes strength.
3. the strength	3. Do you have the strength?
4. there's strength	4. Together there's strength.
5. much strength	5. Does he have much strength?
/skwɛ/	
1. square deal	1. That's a square deal.
2. shoot square	2. He'll shoot square.
3. square peg	3. He's a square peg.
4. square of	4. What's the square of four?
5. square corner	5. Turn a square corner.

/æ/ CONTEXTS

Distinctive features: low-front, lax, unround
/æ/ *consonant combinations:* Initial position of a stressed syllable

Deep Test

/æn/ answer	/æd/ add	/æf/ after	/ækt/ act	/æsk/ ask
/æt/ at	/æk/ action	/æm/ am		

Common Words

/æn/	/æt/	/æd/	/æk/	/æf/	/æm/	/ækt/
animal	at	add	action	after	am	act
answer	attribute					

/æsk/

ask

Everyday Language

Phrases	*Sentences*
/æn/	
1. an answer	1. Give me an answer.
2. answer the	2. Answer the question.
3. animal cracker	3. Want an animal cracker?
4. answer the phone	4. Answer the phone, please.
5. big animal	5. That's a big animal.
/æt/	
1. at home	1. I'll be at home.
2. at school	2. He's at school.
3. at the office	3. She's at the office.
4. at ten	4. We'll start at ten.
5. strongest attribute	5. Her strongest attribute is her looks.
/æd/	
1. add up	1. It doesn't add up.
2. even add	2. Can't you even add?
3. add one	3. Add one more.
4. add it up	4. I'll add it up.
5. it'll add	5. It'll add up to a lot.
/æk/	
1. some action	1. Let's get some action going.
2. the action	2. Stop the action!
3. lot of action	3. There's a lot of action.
4. action games	4. Action games are fun.
5. knee action	5. This one has knee action.
/æf/	
1. after lunch	1. Do it after lunch.
2. after all	2. After all, we're first.
3. after the dance	3. See you after the dance.
4. after you're gone	4. After you're gone, I'll finish.
5. five after	5. It's five after now.

Phrases	*Sentences*
/æm/	
1. am I	1. Am I tired!
2. I am	2. Who says I am?
3. what I am	3. I am what I am!
4. am trying	4. But I am trying!
5. am I supposed	5. Am I supposed to be there?
/ækt/	
1. act your	1. Act your age!
2. an act	2. What an act!
3. on an act	3. Don't put on an act.
4. act two	4. Act Two was best.
5. act like it	5. You don't act like it.
/æsk/	
1. ask me	1. Don't ask me!
2. ask him	2. Ask him first.
3. I ask	3. What should I ask?
4. wanted to ask	4. What you wanted to ask, silly!
5. ask later	5. I'll ask later.

/æ/ CONTEXTS

Distinctive features: low-front, lax, unround
/æ/ ***consonant combinations:*** Initial position of an unstressed syllable

Deep Test

/æk/ accept /æf/ afternoon

Common Words

/æk/	/æf/
accept	afternoon

Everyday Language

Phrases	*Sentences*
/æk/	
1. can't accept	1. I can't accept that.
2. accept it	2. You must accept it.
3. accept less	3. Could you accept less?
4. try to accept	4. I'll try to accept it.
5. at least accept	5. At least accept it gracefully.
/æf/	
1. Wednesday afternoon	1. Come on Wednesday afternoon.
2. afternoon blah's	2. I've got the afternoon blah's.
3. long afternoon	3. This is a long afternoon.
4. afternoon nap	4. I miss my afternoon nap.
5. this afternoon	5. I'm off this afternoon.

/æ/ CONTEXTS

Distinctive features: low front, lax, unround
/æ/ ***consonant combinations:*** Medial position of a stressed syllable

Deep Test

/hæ/ had	/ðæ/ that	/græ/ grass	/tʃæ/ chance
/kæ/ can	/næ/ natural	/stæ/ stand	/præ/ practice
/mæ/ man	/læ/ laugh	/dæ/ dance	/blæ/ black
/bæ/ bad	/gæ/ gather	/θæ/ thank	/bræ/ branch
/pæ/ pass	/ræ/ ran	/sæ/ sat	/træ/ travel
/fæ/ fat	/plæ/ plan	/zæ/ example	/klæ/ class
/væ/ value	/glæ/ glad	/ʃæ/ shall	

Common Words

/hæ/	/kæ/	/mæ/	/bæ/	/fæ/	/pæ/
had	camp	command	back	fact	pass
half	can	demand	bad	family	passage
hand	can't	man	bag	fast	past
hang	cannot	manner	bank	fat	path
happen	captain	marry	battle		
happy	carry	master			
has	catch	matter			
hat	character				
have					
perhaps					

/væ/	/ðæ/	/næ/	/læ/	/gæ/	/ræ/	/plæ/
advance	than	narrow	laugh	began	ran	plan
valley	that	natural	land	gather	rather	plant
value	that's	national	last			

/glæ/	/græ/	/stæ/	/dæ/	/θæ/	/sæ/	/zæ/
glad	grant	stand	dance	thank	sat	example
glass	grass	understand				

/ʃæ/	/tʃæ/	/præ/	/blæ/	/bræ/	/træ/	/klæ/
shall	chance	practice	black	branch	travel	class

Everyday Language

Phrases	*Sentences*
/hæ/	
1. had it	1. I've had it!
2. half bad	2. That wasn't half bad.
3. a hand	3. Give me a hand.
4. happy birthday	4. Happy birthday to you.
5. happen often	5. That doesn't happen often.
/kæ/	
1. camp out	1. Want to camp out?
2. I can't	2. I can't today.
3. catch cold	3. You'll catch cold.
4. can carry	4. It's more than you can carry.
5. oh captain	5. Oh, captain–we're sinking!

Phrases	*Sentences*
/mæ/	
1. man your	1. Man your stations!
2. the command	2. Who gives the command?
3. marry me	3. Will you marry me?
4. the matter	4. What's the matter now?
5. I demand	5. I demand a refund!
/bæ/	
1. it back	1. Give it back.
2. not bad	2. That's not bad.
3. in the bag	3. It's in the bag!
4. bank on it	4. Don't bank on it.
5. that battle	5. We won that battle.
/pæ/	
1. pass the peas	1. Pass the peas, please.
2. last passage	2. Read the last passage.
3. half past	3. It's half past eight.
4. the path	4. Take the path over the bridge.
5. pass right by	5. You'll pass right by it.
/fæ/	
1. known fact	1. It's a known fact.
2. family coming	2. Is your family coming?
3. fast buck	3. Want to make a fast buck?
4. fat chance	4. Fat chance of that.
5. fact of life	5. It's a fact of life.
/væ/	
1. advance the	1. Advance the throttle.
2. advance payment	2. I made an advance payment.
3. in the valley	3. Down in the valley . . .
4. good valley	4. It's a good value.
5. advance quickly	5. He'll advance quickly.
/ðæ/	
1. more than	1. He has more than you.
2. that's true	2. That's true, isn't it?
3. know that	3. I know that.
4. more than that	4. You can't do more than that.
5. that's the way	5. That's the way to go.

Phrases	*Sentences*
/næ/	
1. narrow squeak	1. It was a narrow squeak.
2. national debt	2. It's bigger than the national debt.
3. only natural	3. It's only natural.
4. narrow it	4. Narrow it down to two.
5. first national	5. The First National Bank is closed.
/læ/	
1. don't laugh	1. Don't laugh yet.
2. land the job	2. He may land the job.
3. we're last	3. I'll bet we're last.
4. laugh at	4. Laugh at me, will you!?
5. this land	5. This land is mine.
/gæ/	
1. began here	1. It all began here.
2. I gather	2. I gather you like it.
3. it began	3. It began to rain.
4. gather your	4. Gather your wits about you.
5. she began	5. She began to cry.
/ræ/	
1. I ran	1. I ran my stocking.
2. I'd rather	2. I'd rather die first!
3. she ran	3. She ran a good race.
4. ran out	4. It finally ran out.
5. rather cold	5. Rather cold, isn't it?
/plæ/	
1. good plan	1. That's a good plan.
2. plan first	2. Plan first, then do it.
3. plant your feet	3. Plant your feet firmly.
4. don't plan	4. I don't plan to quit.
5. plant a bigger	5. Plant a bigger garden.
/glæ/	
1. glad for	1. I'm glad for you.
2. glad to	2. Glad to see you!
3. clear as glass	3. It's clear as glass.
4. glass houses	4. People in glass houses _____.
5. glad day	5. This is a glad day for everybody.

Phrases	*Sentences*
/græ/	
1. grant you	1. I grant you that.
2. grass is	2. The grass is always greener!
3. green as grass	3. That's as green as grass!
4. grant permission	4. They won't grant permission.
5. grant applications	5. The grant applications are due.
/stæ/	
1. stand there	1. Don't just stand there!
2. I understand	2. I understand–don't shout!
3. you understand	3. Why can't you understand?
4. stand by	4. Stand by to dive!
5. do understand	5. You do understand, don't you?
/dæ/	
1. to the dance	1. Let's go to the dance.
2. what dance	2. What dance is that?
3. homecoming dance	3. The homecoming dance is tonight.
4. can't dance	4. I can't dance.
5. dance a little	5. Everyone can dance a little.
/θæ/	
1. thank heaven	1. Thank heaven for that!
2. thank you	2. Thank you very much.
3. thank me	3. Don't thank me.
4. thank him	4. Did they thank him?
5. I thank	5. I thank you for that.
/sæ/	
1. sat down	1. He sat down hard.
2. I sat	2. I sat right by her.
3. sat there	3. It sat there for days.
4. sat still	4. She sat still.
5. sat outside	5. We sat outside.
/zæ/	
1. good example	1. Set a good example.
2. one example	2. One example is enough.
3. for example	3. For example, take space.
4. another example	4. Another example is math.
5. bad example	5. He's a bad example.

Phrases	*Sentences*
/ʃæ/	
1. shall we	1. What shall we do?
2. we shall	2. We shall see.
3. shall we go	3. Shall we go in now?
4. I shall	4. I shall ask.
5. shall I	5. Shall I speak up?
/tʃæ/	
1. fat chance	1. Fat chance of that!
2. good chance	2. There's a good chance.
3. take a chance	3. You have to take a chance.
4. can't chance	4. We can't chance losing.
5. one chance	5. It's one chance in a hundred.
/præ/	
1. practice makes	1. Practice makes perfect!
2. you practice	2. When do you practice?
3. I practice	3. I practice two hours every day.
4. practice is	4. Practice is at four.
5. football practice	5. Football practice is over.
/blæ/	
1. black shoes	1. Wear your black shoes.
2. black as night	2. It's as black as night!
3. black or white	3. Black or white—which is it?
4. black is	4. Black is slimming.
5. basic black	5. Wear your basic black dress.
/bræ/	
1. branch out	1. We'll branch out.
2. new branch	2. It's a new branch.
3. which branch	3. Which branch is it?
4. downtown branch	4. It's the downtown branch.
5. left branch	5. Take the left branch.
/træ/	
1. travel often	1. Do you travel often?
2. to travel	2. I love to travel.
3. travel kit	3. Where's my travel kit?
4. travel on	4. Travel on, my friend!
5. you travel	5. You travel too fast.

Phrases	*Sentences*
/klæ/	
1. first class	1. Let's go first class.
2. class of	2. I graduated with the class of ____.
3. my class	3. He's in my class.
4. math class	4. Math class meets first.
5. taking a class	5. Are you taking a class?

/ɑ/ CONTEXTS

Distinctive features: low-back, lax, half-round (unround to half-round)
/ɑ/ ***consonant combinations:*** Initial position of a stressed syllable

Deep Test

/ɑr/ are /ɑn/ honor /ɑrt/ art /ɑrm/ arm

Common Words

/ɑr/	/ɑn/	/ɑrt/	/ɑrm/
are	honor	art	arm
army			
article			

Everyday Language

Phrases	*Sentences*
/ɑr/	
1. are you	1. Are you coming?
2. whole army	2. There's a whole army coming.
3. first article	3. The first article is good.
4. are going	4. We are going, aren't we?
5. who are	5. Who are you going to call?
/ɑn/	
1. my honor	1. On my honor I will.
2. the honor roll	2. Did you make the honor roll?
3. honor your	3. Honor your elders!
4. honor classes	4. He's in honor classes.
5. honor-bound	5. We're honor-bound to do it.

Phrases	*Sentences*
/ɑrt/	
1. pop art	1. Do you like pop art?
2. art class	2. Take an art class.
3. art can	3. Art can be fun.
4. an art	4. It's an art.
5. taking art	5. He's taking art.
/ɑrm/	
1. your arm	1. Raise your arm, please.
2. his arm	2. He broke his arm.
3. right arm	3. I'd give my right arm!
4. arm and a leg	4. It costs an arm and a leg!
5. my arm	5. Take my arm when we cross.

/ɑ/ CONTEXTS

Distinctive features: low-back, lax, half-round (unround to half-round)
/ɑ/ ***consonant combinations:*** Medial position of a stressed syllable

Deep Test

/pɑ/ part	/stɑ/ stop	/nɑ/ not	/rɑ/ rock
/gɑ/ got	/wɑ/ watch	/lɑ/ lot	/drɑ/ drop
/fɑ/ far	/dɑ/ dollar	/jɑ/ beyond	/spɑ/ spot
/kɑ/ car	/hɑ/ hot	/tɑ/ top	/dʒɑ/ job
/mɑ/ modern	/bɑ/ body	/tʃɑ/ charge	
/prɑ/ proper	/ʃɑ/ shop	/hwɑ/ what	

Common Words

/pa/	/ga/	/fa/	/ka/	/ma/	/pra/
department	garden	far	car	march	probable
part	god	farm	college	mark	problem
party	got	farmer	common	market	promise
possible	guard	follow	cotton	modern	proper
upon	regard	following			

/sta/	/wa/	/da/	/ha/	/ba/	/ʃa/	/na/
star	want	dark	heart	body	shop	knowledge
start	wash	doctor	hot	box	shot	not
stock	watch	dollar				
stop						

/la/	/ja/	/ta/	/tʃa/	/hwa/	/ra/	/dra/	/spa/
large	beyond	top	charge	what	rock	drop	spot

/dʒa/
job

Everyday Language

Phrases	*Sentences*
/pa/	
1. men's department	1. Where's the men's department?
2. a part	2. A part is missing.
3. party time	3. It's party time!
4. anything's possible	4. Anything's possible–right?
5. once upon	5. Once upon a time . . .
/ga/	
1. your garden	1. How is your garden doing?
2. my god	2. My god, it's awful!
3. I've got	3. I've got to get help.
4. your guard	4. Your guard is down.
5. I regard	5. I regard him highly.
/fa/	
1. not far	1. It's not far now.
2. who's farm	2. Who's farm is this?
3. a farmer	3. Were you a farmer once?
4. follow directions	4. Just follow directions.
5. I'm following	5. I'm following each step.

Phrases	*Sentences*
/kɑ/	
1. my car	1. My car won't start.
2. at college	2. She's away at college.
3. common cold	3. It's just a common cold.
4. like cotton	4. My head feels like cotton!
5. new car	5. Is that a new car?
/mɑ/	
1. just march	1. Just march in and say so.
2. mark my words	2. Mark my words, she'll go.
3. no market	3. There's no market for it.
4. modern way	4. It's the modern way.
5. mark your place	5. Mark your place here.
/prɑ/	
1. not probable	1. It's possible, not probable.
2. the problem	2. The problem is money.
3. I promise	3. I promise I'll help.
4. only proper	4. It's only proper, you know.
5. such a problem	5. Yes, but it's such a problem.
/stɑ/	
1. the star	1. Who's the star?
2. before you start	2. Think before you start.
3. stock parts	3. We don't stock parts for it.
4. stop by	4. Stop by tonight.
5. can't stop	5. I can't stop tonight.
/wɑ/	
1. want one	1. Do you want one?
2. wash it	2. Wash it first.
3. to watch	3. I can't bear to watch.
4. want you	4. He'll want you to call.
5. watch out	5. Watch out, it's hot!
/dɑ/	
1. it's dark	1. It's dark in here.
2. call the doctor	2. Call the doctor, please.
3. bet a dollar	3. I'll bet a dollar she's here.
4. in the dark	4. We're in the dark.
5. go to doctor	5. Go to Doctor _____.

Phrases	*Sentences*
/hɑ/	
1. my heart	1. My heart just stopped!
2. a heart	2. Have a heart!
3. you're hot	3. When you're hot, you're hot!
4. is it hot	4. Boy, is it hot!
5. heart beat	5. I can feel my heart beat.
/bɑ/	
1. body shop	1. Take it to a body shop.
2. the box	2. Where's the box for it?
3. body beautiful	3. She's the body beautiful!
4. my body	4. My body is tired!
5. in the box	5. It won't fit in the box.
/ʃɑ/	
1. shop around	1. Just shop around for it.
2. long shot	2. It's a long shot.
3. own shop	3. She opened her own shop.
4. he shot	4. He shot two under par.
5. hot shot	5. He tries to be a hot shot.
/nɑ/	
1. little knowledge	1. A little knowledge helps.
2. she's not	2. She's not my type.
3. no knowledge	3. I have no knowledge of that.
4. not ready	4. We're not ready.
5. not going	5. I'm not going.
/lɑ/	
1. one large	1. There's one large one.
2. not a lot	2. That's not a lot.
3. there's a lot	3. There's a lot in a large one.
4. large or small	4. Large or small will do.
5. need a lot	5. We don't need a lot.
/jɑ/	
1. beyond this	1. Beyond this, I doubt it.
2. our yard	2. Come over to our yard.
3. one yard	3. One yard is plenty.
4. beyond this point	4. Don't go beyond this point.
5. beyond me	5. It's beyond me.

Phrases	*Sentences*
/tɑ/	
1. on top	1. He's on top.
2. top of the morning	2. Top of the morning to you!
3. the top to it	3. I lost the top to it.
4. the top	4. This is the top.
5. top it up	5. Top it up a little.
/tʃɑ/	
1. they charge	1. What do they charge?
2. small charge	2. It's a small charge.
3. charge the battery	3. Charge the battery first.
4. charge it	4. Charge it, please.
5. charge card	5. Where's your charge card?
/hwɑ/	
1. what time	1. What time is it?
2. what did	2. What did he say?
3. said what	3. He said what?
4. what she	4. What she said, I think.
5. what is	5. What is the world coming to?
/rɑ/	
1. between a rock	1. We're between a rock and a hard place.
2. hard as rock	2. It's hard as rock.
3. rock 'n roll	3. What happened to "Rock 'N Roll"?
4. rock easy	4. Rock easy in that chair.
5. don't rock	5. Don't rock the boat.
/drɑ/	
1. drop her	1. Drop her a line sometime.
2. drop the ball	2. They may drop the ball.
3. long drop	3. It's a long drop.
4. drop over	4. Drop over sometime.
5. drop in the bucket	5. It's just a drop in the bucket.
/spɑ/	
1. hits the spot	1. That hits the spot.
2. spot on it	2. I got a spot on it.
3. spot one	3. Did you spot one?
4. here spot	4. Here, Spot, here, boy!
5. fun spot	5. That's a fun spot.

Phrases	*Sentences*
/dʒɑ/	
1. get the job	1. Did you get the job?
2. hard job	2. Is it a hard job?
3. a job	3. A job's a job.
4. my job	4. My job is interesting.
5. different job	5. I'd like a different job.

/ɑ/ CONTEXTS

Distinctive features: low-back, lax, half-round (unround to half-round)
/ɑ/ ***consonant combinations:*** Medial position of an unstressed syllable

Deep Test

/hwɑ/ whatever

Common Words

/hwɑ/
whatever

Everyday Language

Phrases	*Sentences*
/hwɑ/	
1. whatever you say	1. Whatever you say, I'll do.
2. whatever happens	2. Whatever happens, we're friends
3. whatever happened	3. Whatever happened to her?
4. whatever I say	4. Whatever I say, it's wrong.
5. whatever shall	5. Whatever shall we do?

/ɑ/ CONTEXTS

Distinctive features: low-back, lax, half-round (unround to half-round)
/ɑ/ ***consonant combinations:*** Final position of a stressed syllable

Deep Test

/fɑ/ father

Common Words

/fɑ/

father

Everyday Language

Phrases	*Sentences*
/fɑ/	
1. my father	1. My father is coming.
2. the father	2. The father of our country was _____.
3. your father	3. Ask your father.
4. father's day	4. Father's Day is _____.
5. like your father	5. You look like your father.

/ɔ/ CONTEXTS

Distinctive features: low-mid-back, lax, round
/ɔ/ ***consonant combinations:*** Initial position of a stressed syllable

Deep Test

/ɔf/ off   /ɔl/ all   /ɔr/ or

Common Words

/ɔf/	/ɔl/	/ɔr/
off	all	or
offer	almost	order
office	also	
officer	always	
often		

Everyday Language

Phrases	*Sentences*
/ɔf/	
1. good offer	1. That's a good offer.
2. her office	2. Where's her office?
3. very often	3. I don't go very often.
4. offer him	4. Offer him some help.
5. day off	5. Tomorrow is my day off.

Phrases	*Sentences*
/ɔl/	
1. all over	1. It's all over.
2. almost finished	2. He's almost finished.
3. also need	3. You'll also need a pen.
4. always rains	4. It always rains on Monday.
5. almost always	5. Well, almost always.
/ɔr/	
1. right or wrong	1. You're either right or wrong.
2. let's order	2. Let's order a sandwich.
3. big order	3. That's a big order.
4. you or me	4. It's you or me!
5. a little order	5. Let's have a little order!

/ɔ/ CONTEXTS

Distinctive features: low-mid-back, lax, round
/ɔ/ ***consonant combinations:*** Initial position of an unstressed syllable

Deep Test

/ɔl/ although

Common Words

/ɔl/

already
although

Everyday Language

Phrases	*Sentences*
/ɔl/	
1. already done	1. It's already done.
2. although I can't	2. I'll try, although I can't be sure.
3. once already	3. He's been told once already.
4. already late	4. We're already late.
5. although it's raining	5. Although it's raining, we'll go.

/ɔ/ CONTEXTS

Distinctive features: low-mid-back, lax, round
/ɔ/ ***consonant combinations:*** Medial position of a stressed syllable

Deep Test

/kɔ/ call	/tɔ/ tall	/dɔ/ dog	/kwɔ/ quarter
/fɔ/ fall	/krɔ/ across	/gɔ/ gone	/stɔ/ storm
/lɔ/ along	/hɔ/ hall	/θɔ/ thought	/smɔ/ small
/wɔ/ wall	/nɔ/ north	/ʃɔ/ short	/strɔ/ destroy
/sɔ/ song	/pɔ/ important	/rɔ/ wrong	
/mɔ/ morning	/bɔ/ born	/brɔ/ brought	

Common Words

/kɔ/	/fɔ/	/lɔ/	/wɔ/	/sɔ/	/mɔ/	/tɔ/
according	fall	along	walk	salt	morning	talk
because	for	belong	wall	song	tomorrow	tall
call	forest	long	war	short		
caught	foreign	lord	warm			
cause	form	loss				
corner	former	lost				
cost	forward					

/krɔ/	/hɔ/	/nɔ/	/pɔ/	/bɔ/	/dɔ/	/gɔ/
across	hall	north	important	born	dog	gone
cross	horse					

/θɔ/	/ʃɔ/	/rɔ/	/brɔ/	/kwɔ/	/stɔ/	/smɔ/
thought	short	wrong	brought	quarter	storm	small

/strɔ/
strong

Everyday Language

Phrases	*Sentences*
/kɔ/	
1. according to this	1. According to this, we won.
2. that's because	2. That's because we're best.
3. I'd call	3. I'd call that class!
4. caught up	4. We finally caught up.
5. around the corner	5. It's just around the corner.

Phrases	*Sentences*
/fɔ/	
1. like fall	1. I like fall best.
2. one for me	2. One for me, one for you!
3. a form	3. Did you fill out a form?
4. former teacher	4. She's a former teacher.
5. step forward	5. It's a step forward.
/lɔ/	
1. belong here	1. We don't belong here.
2. walk along	2. Let's walk along the tracks.
3. long way	3. It's a long way yet.
4. small loss	4. It's a small loss.
5. who lost	5. If we won, who lost?
/wɔ/	
1. take a walk	1. Let's take a walk.
2. the wall	2. I'm climbing the wall!
3. war on	3. There's a war on now.
4. nice and warm	4. It's nice and warm.
5. walk faster	5. Walk faster, please.
/sɔ/	
1. her salt	1. She's worth her salt.
2. salt and pepper	2. Pass the salt and pepper.
3. great song	3. That's a great song!
4. sort it out	4. We can't sort it out.
5. some sort	5. He's a teacher of some sort.
/mɔ/	
1. good morning	1. Have a good morning!
2. tomorrow morning	2. Tomorrow morning will be fine.
3. 'til tomorrow	3. Put it off 'til tomorrow.
4. morning is	4. Morning is the best time.
5. morning comes	5. Morning comes so early!
/tɔ/	
1. talk, talk	1. Talk, talk–that's all you do!
2. he's tall	2. He's tall for his age.
3. talk back	3. Don't talk back.
4. tall girls	4. Tall girls are pretty.
5. let's talk	5. Let's talk about it.

Phrases	*Sentences*
/krɔ/	
1. two across	1. Move two across and one down.
2. cross the street	2. Cross the street carefully.
3. came across	3. I came across it yesterday.
4. make a cross	4. Make a cross here.
5. cross me up	5. Don't cross me up.
/hɔ/	
1. down the hall	1. Down the hall and to the left.
2. ride a horse	2. Can you ride a horse?
3. end of the hall	3. It's at the end of the hall.
4. horse around	4. Boys like to horse around.
5. like a horse	5. He eats like a horse!
/nɔ/	
1. go north	1. Go north two blocks.
2. live up north	2. Would you live up north?
3. north of here	3. It's north of here.
4. north, south, east	4. North, south, east, west, _____ is best!
5. North Star	5. Can you see the North Star?
/pɔ/	
1. important message	1. Here's an important message.
2. feel important	2. Don't you feel important?
3. important people	3. We're important people.
4. be important	4. It could be important.
5. it's important	5. She says it's important.
/bɔ/	
1. born tired	1. I was born tired!
2. born yesterday	2. He wasn't born yesterday.
3. were you born	3. Where were you born?
4. was born	4. I was born at home.
5. born loser	5. You're a born loser!
/dɔ/	
1. dog's life	1. It's a dog's life!
2. good dog	2. Be a good dog!
3. hot dog	3. How about a hot dog?
4. doggone	4. Doggone, we won!
5. dirty dog	5. You dirty dog!

Phrases	*Sentences*
/gɔ/	
1. all gone	1. It's all gone.
2. already gone	2. He's already gone.
3. long gone	3. She's long gone!
4. been gone	4. How long have they been gone?
5. were gone	5. We were gone two weeks.
/θɔ/	
1. thought so	1. I thought so.
2. thought that	2. Who'd have thought that?
3. thought about	3. I thought about you a lot.
4. good thought	4. That's a good thought.
5. thought it over	5. She thought it over.
/ʃɔ/	
1. we're short	1. We're short on chairs.
2. too short	2. You're too short.
3. short or tall	3. Short or tall, I like you.
4. long and short	4. That's the long and short of it.
5. short people	5. Short people think big.
/rɔ/	
1. what's wrong	1. What's wrong now?
2. nothing's wrong	2. Nothing's wrong at all.
3. you're wrong	3. I'll bet you're wrong.
4. right or wrong	4. Right or wrong, it's OK.
5. wrong with	5. What's wrong with you?
/brɔ/	
1. brought you	1. Who brought you home?
2. we brought	2. We brought a present.
3. brought a friend	3. She brought a friend.
4. Bill brought	4. Bill brought Amy.
5. brought his	5. Sam brought his dog.
/kwɔ/	
1. it's a quarter	1. It's a quarter past eight.
2. a quarter	2. Lend me a quarter.
3. you a quarter	3. I'll bet you a quarter.
4. in a quarter	4. There are _____ nickles in a quarter.
5. quarterback	5. Who plays quarterback?

Phrases	*Sentences*
/stɔ/	
1. up a storm	1. She kicked up a storm!
2. storm is coming	2. Looks like a storm is coming.
3. storm warning	3. The storm warning is out.
4. hear the storm	4. Did you hear the storm last night?
5. what storm	5. What storm was that?
/smɔ/	
1. small world	1. It's a small world!
2. small one	2. Take the small one.
3. small cars	3. Small cars are fun.
4. be small	4. Don't be small about it.
5. small thing	5. It's a small thing.
/strɔ/	
1. you strong	1. Are you strong?
2. strong people	2. We need strong people.
3. strong coffee	3. That's strong coffee.
4. strong rope	4. A strong rope will hold it.
5. strong medicine	5. That's strong medicine.

/ɔ/ CONTEXTS

Distinctive features: low-mid-back, lax, round
/ɔ/ ***consonant combinations:*** Final position of a stressed syllable

Deep Test

/sɔ/ saw   /dɔ/ daughter   /lɔ/ law   /drɔ/ draw

Common Words

/sɔ/	/dɔ/	/lɔ/	/drɔ/
saw	daughter	law	draw
soft			

Everyday Language

Phrases	*Sentences*
/sɔ/	
1. I saw	1. I saw it first.
2. she saw	2. She saw it too.
3. saw it	3. If I saw it, it's mine.
4. who saw	4. It doesn't matter who saw it first.
5. too soft	5. You're too soft.
/dɔ/	
1. your daughter	1. Is this your daughter?
2. second daughter	2. She's my second daughter.
3. one daughter	3. Do you have more than one daughter?
4. oldest daughter	4. My oldest daughter is away.
5. youngest daughter	5. This is my youngest daughter.
/lɔ/	
1. the law	1. It's the law, you know.
2. broke the law	2. Who broke the law?
3. made the law	3. Who made the law?
4. which law	4. Which law do you mean?
5. Murphy's Law	5. Have you heard of Murphy's Law?
/drɔ/	
1. draw up	1. Let's draw up a plan.
2. draw animals	2. Can you draw animals?
3. draw anything	3. He can draw anything.
4. draw the line	4. That's where I draw the line!
5. draw a card	5. OK, now draw a card.

/o/ CONTEXTS

Distinctive features: high-mid-back, tense, round
/o/ *consonant combinations:* Initial position of a stressed syllable

Deep Test

/o/ open   /on/ only   /old/ old

Common Words

/o/	/on/	/old/
ocean	only	old
oh	own	
open		
over		

Everyday Language

Phrases	*Sentences*
/o/	
1. ocean blue	1. Sail the ocean blue!
2. oh there	2. Oh, there you are!
3. open the door	3. Open the door, please.
4. all over	4. It's all over now.
5. I'm open	5. I'm open to suggestion.
/on/	
1. only money	1. It's only money.
2. own one	2. Do you own one?
3. only kidding	3. I'm only kidding.
4. own car	4. I have my own car.
5. only three	5. There are only three left.
/old/	
1. old business	1. Any old business?
2. old story	2. That's an old story.
3. old friends	3. Old friends are best.
4. old one	4. Don't worry, it's an old one.
5. old injury	5. It's caused by an old injury.

/o/ CONTEXTS

Distinctive features: high-mid-back, tense, round
/o/ ***consonant combinations:*** Medial position of a stressed syllable

Deep Test

/ko/ coat	/so/ soul	/klo/ close	/wo/ won't
/ho/ hole	/no/ note	/sto/ store	/bro/ broken
/po/ post	/to/ told	/vo/ vote	/tro/ control
/ro/ road	/do/ don't	/ðo/ those	/flo/ floor
/fo/ before	/go/ gold	/mo/ most	/spo/ spoke
/bo/ boat	/ʃo/ shoulder	/lo/ alone	/smo/ smoke

Common Words

/ko/	/ho/	/po/	/ro/	/fo/	/bo/	/so/
coal	hold	post	road	before	board	sold
coat	hole	report	rose	force	boat	soldier
cold	home	support	roll	four	both	soul
course	hope	suppose	wrote			
court	whole					

/no/	/to/	/do/	/go/	/ʃo/	/klo/	/sto/
known	told	don't	gold	shore	close	stone
nose	toward	door	golden	shoulder	clothes	store
note						

/vo/	/ðo/	/mo/	/lo/	/wo/	/bro/	/tro/	/flo/
vote	those	most	alone	won't	broken	control	floor

/spo/	/smo/
spoke	smoke

Everyday Language

Phrases	***Sentences***
/ko/	
1. black as coal	1. It was black as coal.
2. new coat	2. Is that a new coat?
3. it's cold	3. It's cold in here.
4. of course	4. Of course she will.
5. in court	5. It's your day in court.

Phrases	*Sentences*
/ho/	
1. get hold	1. Get hold of yourself.
2. in the hole	2. We're in the hole now.
3. be home	3. It's good to be home.
4. I hope	4. I hope you can.
5. the whole thing	5. He ate the whole thing.
/po/	
1. post office	1. Is the post office open?
2. long report	2. That's a long report.
3. our support	3. They'll need our support.
4. I suppose	4. I suppose they will.
5. report to work	5. Report to work at eight.
/ro/	
1. which road	1. Which road do we take?
2. a rose	2. A rose between two thorns!
3. roll and coffee	3. I'd like a roll and coffee.
4. who wrote	4. Who wrote this book?
5. I wrote	5. I wrote him a note.
/fo/	
1. before beauty	1. Age before beauty!
2. police force	2. He joined the police force.
3. is four	3. Two times two is four.
4. before	4. We were here before you.
5. use force	5. There's no need to use force.
/bo/	
1. room and board	1. You get room and board.
2. missed the boat	2. We missed the boat!
3. both of us	3. Both of us can work.
4. new board	4. It'll take a new board.
5. both hands	5. Use both hands.
/so/	
1. sold out	1. They're sold out.
2. my soul	2. Bless my soul!
3. sold my car	3. I sold my car.
4. soldier now	4. Is he a soldier now?
5. soul mate	5. She's my soul mate.

Phrases	*Sentences*
/no/	
1. isn't known	1. Just how many isn't known.
2. your nose	2. Don't put your nose in!
3. a note	3. Send a note.
4. note the	4. Note the fine detail.
5. punch your nose	5. He'll punch your nose!
/to/	
1. told you	1. I told you so.
2. step toward	2. It's a step toward the end.
3. toward the door	3. Move toward the door.
4. told it	4. They told it over and over.
5. told a lie	5. He told a lie.
/do/	
1. don't mention	1. Don't mention it.
2. don't tell	2. Don't tell me!
3. the door	3. Open the door.
4. don't know	4. I don't know.
5. the door is	5. The door is always open.
/go/	
1. gold mine	1. It's a gold mine.
2. golden opportunity	2. It's a golden opportunity.
3. isn't gold	3. All that glitters isn't gold.
4. kind of gold	4. It turned kind of gold-colored.
5. golden hair	5. She has golden hair.
/ʃo/	
1. the shore	1. I love the shore.
2. need a shoulder	2. I need a shoulder to cry on.
3. shoreline is	3. The shoreline is lovely.
4. soft shoulder	4. Watch the soft shoulder!
5. shoulder the	5. Shoulder the load!
/klo/	
1. close up	1. They close up late.
2. nice clothes	2. What nice clothes!
3. close the door	3. Close the door, please.
4. clothes make	4. Clothes make the man.
5. clothes horse	5. She's a clothes horse.

Phrases	*Sentences*
/sto/	
1. throw stones	1. Don't throw stones.
2. at the store	2. Stop at the store, please.
3. hard as stone	3. It's hard as stone.
4. store it up	4. Store it up for winter.
5. stone's throw	5. It's a stone's throw.
/vo/	
1. for the vote	1. Call for the vote.
2. vote yes	2. The aye's vote "Yes."
3. vote no	3. The nay's vote "No."
4. you vote	4. Did you vote?
5. vote for it	5. I vote for it.
/ðo/	
1. those are	1. Those are fine.
2. are those	2. Whose are those?
3. those fit	3. Those fit well.
4. those people	4. Those people can.
5. those books	5. I gave her those books.
/mo/	
1. most of the time	1. Most of the time it works.
2. like most	2. Which do you like most?
3. red the most	3. I like red the most.
4. most people	4. Most people don't.
5. not most people	5. Well, I'm not most people!
/lo/	
1. alone today	1. She's alone today.
2. go alone	2. I can go alone.
3. better alone	3. It's better alone.
4. be alone	4. It's good to be alone.
5. all alone	5. We're all alone now.
/wo/	
1. won't tell	1. He won't tell.
2. won't go	2. We won't go.
3. won't you	3. Won't you, please?
4. won't fit	4. It won't fit.
5. won't find	5. You won't find it.

Phrases	*Sentences*
/bro/	
1. broken again	1. It's broken again.
2. always broken	2. It's always broken.
3. we've broken	3. We've broken it twice.
4. broken parts	4. Broken parts won't work.
5. broken heads	5. Broken heads won't either!
/tro/	
1. lost control	1. He lost control.
2. the control	2. Here's the control.
3. control it	3. Control it now!
4. one control	4. One control is enough.
5. some control	5. We need some control.
/flo/	
1. the floor	1. You have the floor.
2. floor me	2. You floor me!
3. on the floor	3. She's flat on the floor.
4. floor sample	4. Here's a floor sample.
5. first floor	5. The first floor is best.
/spo/	
1. spoke first	1. I spoke first.
2. never spoke	2. She never spoke.
3. we spoke	3. We spoke our piece!
4. spoke well	4. They spoke well of her.
5. one spoke	5. One spoke is broken.
/smo/	
1. there's smoke	1. Where there's smoke, _____.
2. you smoke	2. Do you smoke?
3. smoke a pipe	3. I smoke a pipe.
4. pipe smoke	4. I hate pipe smoke.
5. smell smoke	5. I smell smoke!

/o/ CONTEXTS

Distinctive features: high-mid-back, tense, round
/o/ ***consonant combinations:*** Medial position of an unstressed syllable

Deep Test

/mo/ almost /ro/ railroad

Common Words

/mo/	/ro/
almost	railroad

Everyday Language

Phrases	*Sentences*
/mo/	
1. almost any	1. Almost any time now!
2. almost ready	2. They're almost ready.
3. almost everyone	3. Almost everyone does.
4. almost missed	4. He almost missed.
5. almost fits	5. It almost fits.
/ro/	
1. at the railroad	1. Stop at the railroad.
2. railroad it	2. We can railroad it through.
3. to the railroad	3. Let's walk to the railroad.
4. railroad crossing	4. There's a railroad crossing.
5. railroad trip	5. A railroad trip is fun.

/o/ CONTEXTS

Distinctive features: high-mid-back, tense, round
/o/ ***consonant combinations:*** Final position of a stressed syllable

Deep Test

/go/ ago	/ðo/ though	/mo/ moment	/sto/ story
/no/ no	/so/ so	/gro/ grow	/sno/ snow
/lo/ low	/ʃo/ show	/flo/ flow	

Common Words

/go/	/no/	/lo/	/ðo/	/so/	/ʃo/	/mo/	/gro/
ago	know	below	although	so	show	moment	grow
go	no	low					
going	notice	lower					

/flo/	/sto/	/sno/
flow	story	snow

Everyday Language

Phrases	*Sentences*
/go/	
1. long time ago	1. That was a long time ago.
2. go along	2. Go along with me, OK?
3. I'm going	3. I'm going to try.
4. go ahead	4. Go ahead, do it!
5, two years ago	5. We started two years ago.
/no/	
1. no use	1. It's no use.
2. a notice	2. Put up a notice
3. know it	3. I know it.
4. no way	4. There's no way out.
5. no one	5. No one knows.
/lo/	
1. below zero	1. It's below zero.
2. low blow	2. That's a low blow.
3. lower level	3. Try the lower level.
4. down below	4. What's down below?
5. low price	5. That's a low price.
/ðo/	
1. although she won't	1. I'll go although she won't.
2. would though	2. She said she would, though.
3. although it's late	3. Although it's late, we'll take it.
4. even though	4. We should, even though it's hard.
5. though you	5. It's alright even though you promised.

Phrases	*Sentences*
/so/	
1. so what	1. He just said, "So what?"
2. so long	2. It's been so long.
3. so there	3. So there, you do it.
4. told you so	4. I told you so.
5. so tired	5. I'm so tired.
/ʃo/	
1. show up	1. He didn't show up.
2. show me	2. Show me how.
3. good show	3. Good show, team!
4. show me up	4. Don't show me up!
5. show starts	5. The show starts soon.
/mo/	
1. a moment	1. Wait a moment!
2. in a moment	2. In a moment we will.
3. only a moment	3. Only a moment to go.
4. one more moment	4. One more moment; then start.
5. a moment more	5. A moment more and I'd have died!
/gro/	
1. grow up	1. Please grow up!
2. grow on you	2. It will grow on you.
3. garden grow	3. How does your garden grow?
4. grow flowers	4. Can you grow flowers?
5. grow fast	5. It'll grow fast.
/flo/	
1. flow along	1. It'll flow along.
2. flow by	2. Time will flow by.
3. seems to flow	3. Her hair seems to flow!
4. seemed to flow	4. The words seemed to flow.
5. flow chart	5. Let's make a flow chart.
/sto/	
1. tall story	1. That's a tall story!
2. your story	2. What's your story?
3. story to	3. There's a story behind this.
4. four story	4. It's a four story building.
5. different story	5. That's a different story.

Phrases	*Sentences*
/sno/	
1. like snow	1. Do you like snow?
2. white as snow	2. It's white as snow.
3. snow job	3. What a snow job!
4. it will snow	4. Do you think it will snow?
5. snow plow	4. Where's the snow plow?

/o/ CONTEXTS

Distinctive features: high-mid-back, tense, round
/o/ *consonant combinations:* Final position of an unstressed syllable

Deep Test

/do/ window /so/ also

Common Words

/do/	/so/
window	also

Everyday Language

Phrases	*Sentences*
/do/	
1. the window	1. Open the window.
2. by the window	2. Stand by the window.
3. in the window	3. It's in the window.
4. which window	4. Which window is yours?
5. washed the window	5. Who washed the window?
/so/	
1. mine also	1. Take mine also.
2. also came	2. She also came.
3. problem also	3. That's a problem also.
4. to do also	4. There's a job to do also.
5. also we need	5. Also, we need to hurry.

/ᴜ/ CONTEXTS

Distinctive features: high-back, lax, round
/ᴜ/ ***consonant combinations:*** Medial position of a stressed syllable

Deep Test

/kᴜ/ cook	/pᴜ/ put	/fᴜ/ foot	/tᴜ/ took	/lᴜ/ look
/ʃᴜ/ should	/jᴜ/ you're	/bᴜ/ book	/gᴜ/ good	/stᴜ/ stood
/wᴜ/ wood				

Common Words

/kᴜ/	/ʃᴜ/	/wᴜ/	/pᴜ/	/jᴜ/	/fᴜ/	/bᴜ/
cook	should	woman	pull	you're	foot	book
could	sugar	wood	put	your	full	
couldn't	sure	would				

/tᴜ/	/gᴜ/	/lᴜ/	/stᴜ/
took	good	look	stood

Everyday Language

Phrases	*Sentences*
/kᴜ/	
1. great cook	1. She's a great cook.
2. you cook	2. Can you cook?
3. the cookbook	3. Where's the cookbook?
4. couldn't tell	4. I couldn't tell you.
5. you could	5. You could if you would.
/ʃᴜ/	
1. should be going	1. I should be going.
2. the sugar	2. Pass the sugar.
3. sure hope	3. I sure hope so.
4. you should	4. You should tell me.
5. you sure	5. Are you sure?
/wᴜ/	
1. a woman	1. That's a woman for you!
2. wood is	2. Wood is pretty.
3. would you	3. Would you be willing?
4. good woman	4. She's a good woman.
5. like wood	5. I like wood best.

Phrases	*Sentences*
/pʊ/	
1. don't pull	1. Don't pull too hard.
2. put out	2. Put out your hand.
3. lot of pull	3. He has a lot of pull.
4. put up	4. Put up or _____.
5. pull out	5. You can pull out now.
/jʊ/	
1. you're too good	1. You're too good for me.
2. your turn	2. It's your turn.
3. your way	3. Your way is best.
4. you're telling	4. You're telling me!
5. you're not	5. You're not going?
/fʊ/	
1. best foot	1. Put your best foot forward.
2. full time	2. It's a full time job.
3. full one	3. I'd like a full one.
4. tank full	4. One tank full should do it.
5. foot long	5. It's about a foot long.
/bʊ/	
1. write a book	1. Could you write a book?
2. book a room	2. Better book a room early.
3. wrote the book	3. Who wrote the book?
4. good book	4. It's a good book.
5. her book	5. I'll borrow her book.
/tʊ/	
1. it took	1. It took a long time.
2. we took	2. We took two days.
3. took me	3. It took me by surprise.
4. he took	4. He took the course.
5. took two	5. It took two of us.
/gʊ/	
1. good time	1. What a good time!
2. good day	2. Have a good day!
3. good bye	3. Good bye, old friend!
4. good morning	4. Good morning, all!
5. it's good	5. It's good to see you.

Phrases	*Sentences*
/lʊ/	
1. one look	1. I took one look.
2. look here	2. Look here now!
3. look up	3. Look up here, please.
4. you look	4. You look great!
5. look straight	5. Look straight ahead.
/stʊ/	
1. she stood	1. She stood by me.
2. it stood	2. There it stood.
3. it stood all	3. It stood all alone.
4. I stood	4. I stood it as long as I could.
5. we stood	5. We stood for two hours.

/ʊ/ CONTEXTS

Distinctive features: high-back, lax, round
/ʊ/ ***consonant combinations:*** Medial position of an unstressed syllable

Deep Test

/ʒʊ/ usually /jʊ/ yourself

Common Words

/ʒʊ/	/jʊ/
usually	yourself

Everyday Language

Phrases	*Sentences*
/ʒʊ/	
1. usually rains	1. It usually rains.
2. usually stay	2. We usually stay home.
3. usually play	3. They usually play well.
4. usually we	4. Usually we don't.
5. usually busy	5. Are you usually busy?

Phrases	*Sentences*
/jʊ/	
1. do it yourself	1. Do it yourself, then.
2. for yourself	2. Save one for yourself.
3. for yourself then	3. See for yourself, then.
4. besides yourself	4. Who's going besides yourself?
5. beside yourself	5. You'll be beside yourself.

/u/ CONTEXTS

Distinctive features: high-back, tense, round
/u/ ***consonant combinations:*** Medial position of a stressed syllable

Deep Test

/mu/ moon	/hu/ whom	/lu/ lose	/gru/ group
/ju/ use	/nju/ news	/pru/ prove	/fju/ refuse
/ru/ rule	/bju/ beauty	/tru/ truth	/fru/ fruit
/fu/ food	/ku/ cool	/dju/ produce	/sku/ school
/su/ soon	/nu/ afternoon	/klu/ include	/mju/ music

Common Words

/mu/	/ju/	/ru/	/fu/	/su/	/hu/	/nju/
moon	union	rule	food	soon	whom	news
move	use	roof	fool	suit	whose	newspaper
movement	youth	room				
remove						

/bju/	/ku/	/nu/	/lu/	/pru/	/tru/	/dju/
beauty	cool	afternoon	lose	prove	truth	produce

/klu/	/gru/	/fju/	/fru/	/sku/	/mju/
include	group	refuse	fruit	school	music

Everyday Language

Phrases	*Sentences*
/mu/	
1. new moon	1. There's a new moon.
2. move over	2. Move over, please.
3. the movement	3. Join the movement now.
4. remove ink	4. How do you remove ink?
5. move now	5. We have to move now.
/ju/	
1. join the union	1. Did you join the union?
2. use some	2. I could use some.
3. youth group	3. How big is the youth group.
4. use it all	4. Did you use it all?
5. union help	5. Will a union help?
/ru/	
1. the rule	1. What's the rule?
2. raise the roof	2. Let's raise the roof.
3. my room	3. Come to my room.
4. a rule	4. Is there a rule?
5. be room	5. There won't be room.
/fu/	
1. enough food	1. There's enough food.
2. fool me	2. You can't fool me.
3. food for thought	3. It's food for thought.
4. no fool	4. He's no fool.
5. food sounds	5. Food sounds good.
/su/	
1. come as soon	1. Come as soon as you can.
2. suit you	2. Does that suit you?
3. soon be over	3. It'll soon be over.
4. soon know	4. We'll soon know.
5. suit yourself	5. Suit yourself, I guess!
/hu/	
1. to whom	1. To whom should I give it?
2. whose book	2. Whose book is this?
3. whose place	3. Whose place will you take?
4. for whom	4. For whom did they ask?
5. whose problem	5. Whose problem is it?

Phrases	*Sentences*
/nju/	
1. hear the news	1. Did you hear the news?
2. in the newspaper	2. I saw it in the newspaper.
3. not new	3. That's not new, is it?
4. no news	4. No news is good news.
5. the newspaper will	5. The newspaper will have it.
/bju/	
1. a beauty	1. Now that's a beauty!
2. beautiful person	2. You're a beautiful person.
3. beautiful night	3. It's a beautiful night.
4. real beauty	4. You can tell real beauty.
5. beauty of it	5. That's the real beauty of it.
/ku/	
1. cool it	1. Alright, cool it!
2. stay cool	2. Just stay cool.
3. cool weather	3. Cool weather is coming.
4. cool off	4. It'll cool off soon.
5. cool off first	5. Let him cool off first.
/nu/	
1. this afternoon	1. Come over this afternoon.
2. tomorrow afternoon	2. Tomorrow afternoon is better.
3. afternoon nap	3. I miss my afternoon nap.
4. afternoon is	4. Afternoon is better than morning.
5. this afternoon for sure	5. Let's make it at one this afternoon
/lu/	
1. you lose	1. Gin, you lose.
2. he lose	2. Did he lose?
3. lose again	3. Well, we lose again!
4. win or lose	4. Win or lose, it's fun.
5. born to lose	5. She's born to lose.
/pru/	
1. prove it	1. OK, prove it.
2. can't prove it	2. I can't prove it.
3. have to prove	3. You have to prove it.
4. why prove	4. Why prove it?
5. prove it if	5. Prove it if you can.

Phrases	*Sentences*
/tru/	
1. that's the truth	1. Now that's the truth.
2. the truth	2. What's the truth?
3. it's the truth	3. It's the truth about her.
4. know it's the truth	4. How do you know it's the truth?
5. only the truth	5. Only the truth matters.
/dju/	
1. produce the goods	1. Can he produce the goods?
2. expensive to produce	2. It's expensive to produce.
3. have to produce	3. You have to produce.
4. if you produce	4. If you produce, it will pay.
5. produce more	5. We can produce more.
/klu/	
1. include tax	1. Does that include tax?
2. include me	2. Will you include me?
3. include postage	3. Include postage, too.
4. include mine	4. Include mine with the rest.
5. include everyone	5. The list will include everyone.
/gru/	
1. join the group	1. Let's join the group.
2. good group	2. It's a good group.
3. in the group	3. Who's in the group.
4. of the group	4. We'll be part of the group.
5. group work	5. Group work is fine.
/fju/	
1. I refuse	1. I refuse to do it.
2. you refuse	2. Why should you refuse?
3. refuse to be	3. Because I refuse to be alone.
4. refuse you	4. Did we refuse you?
5. still refuse	5. I still refuse, so there!
/fru/	
1. fresh fruit	1. I love fresh fruit.
2. what fruit	2. What fruit is in season?
3. fruit are ready	3. All kinds of fruit are ready.
4. fruit salad	4. How about some fruit salad?
5. fruit cup	5. A fruit cup would be good.

Phrases	*Sentences*
/sku/	
1. is school	1. When is school over?
2. school just	2. School just started.
3. like school	3. I like school.
4. school can be	4. School can be fun.
5. school can be long	5. School can be long, too.
/mju/	
1. there's music	1. There's music in the air!
2. some music	2. Let's have some music.
3. beautiful music	3. This is beautiful music.
4. that's music	4. That's music to my ears.
5. music major	5. She's a music major.

/u/ CONTEXTS

Distinctive features: high-back, tense, round
/u/ ***consonant combinations:*** Medial position of an unstressed syllable

Deep Test

/bju/ attribute

Common Words

/bju/
attrìbute

Everyday Language

Phrases	*Sentences*
/bju/	
1. good attribute	1. That's a good attribute.
2. attribute your success	2. To what do you attribute your success?
3. attribute it	3. I attribute it to brains.
4. I attribute	4. I attribute it to hard work.
5. an attribute	5. Brains are an attribute, alright.

/u/ CONTEXTS

Distinctive features: high-back, tense, round
/u/ ***consonant combinations:*** Final position of a stressed syllable

Deep Test

/tu/ to	/fju/ few	/ʃu/ shoe	/tru/ true	/θru/ through
/du/ do	/nu/ new	/hju/ human	/gru/ grew	/hu/ who
/bju/ beauty	/ju/ usually	/blu/ blue	/vju/ view	/mju/ music

Common Words

/tu/	/du/	/bju/	/fju/	/nu/	/ju/	/ʃu/
to	do	beautiful	few	knew	usually	shoe
too	due	beauty	future	new		
two	duty					

/hju/	/blu/	/tru/	/gru/	/vju/	/θru/	/hu/	/mju/
human	blue	true	grew	view	through	who	music

Everyday Language

Phrases	***Sentences***
/tu/	
1. to work	1. He went to work.
2. went too	2. She went too.
3. two days	3. We'll have two days.
4. too many	4. That's not too many.
5. to go	5. It's time to go.
/du/	
1. do it	1. I'll do it.
2. she do it	2. Will she do it?
3. do it every time	3. They'll do it every time.
4. they do it	4. When did they do it?
5. they do	5. What did they do?
/bju/	
1. beautiful day	1. What a beautiful day!
2. real beauty	2. It's a real beauty.
3. brains and beauty	3. She has brains and beauty.
4. beautiful people	4. They're beautiful people.
5. beauty surrounds	5. Beauty surrounds us!

Phrases	*Sentences*
/fju/	
1. few people	1. Few people really know.
2. in the future	2. What's in the future?
3. the future	3. The future is uncertain.
4. a few things	4. I know a few things.
5. a few	5. A few is better than none.
/nu/	
1. knew it	1. I knew it would happen.
2. what's new	2. So what's new about that?
3. nothing new	3. It's nothing new.
4. knew about it	4. He knew about it.
5. new idea	5. It's a new idea.
/ju/	
1. usually open	1. They're usually open.
2. usually know	2. We usually know in advance.
3. usually rains	3. It usually rains.
4. usually home	4. Are you usually home?
5. usually lose	5. They usually lose.
/ʃu/	
1. shoe fits	1. If the shoe fits, _____.
2. throw a shoe	2. Don't throw a shoe!
3. this shoe	3. Try on this shoe.
4. new shoe	4. A new shoe is tight.
5. other shoe	5. Well, drop the other shoe!
/hju/	
1. only human	1. She's only human.
2. is human	2. To err is human, _____.
3. human dignity	3. Human dignity is important.
4. human anatomy	4. Did you take Human Anatomy?
5. human body	5. The human body is mysterious.
/blu/	
1. a blue mood	1. I'm in a blue mood.
2. blue is	2. Blue is my favorite color.
3. blue moon	3. We go once in a blue moon.
4. was blue	4. The air was blue!
5. blue smoke	5. Watch for blue smoke.

Phrases	*Sentences*
/tru/	
1. true or false	1. Is it true or false?
2. true friend	2. Be a true friend.
3. really true	3. What's really true?
4. true to me	4. She's true to me.
5. true love	5. True love never dies!
/gru/	
1. grew on me	1. It just grew on me.
2. grew up	2. It grew up over night.
3. grew several	3. We grew several plants.
4. we grew	4. We grew to know him.
5. they grew	5. They grew up together.
/vju/	
1. my view	1. That's my view.
2. good view	2. Is there a good view?
3. view it first	3. View it first; then tell me.
4. I view	4. I view it as wrong.
5. point of view	5. That's your point of view.
/θru/	
1. through now	1. We're through now.
2. through and through	2. It's rotten through and through.
3. through thick and thin	3. We're together through thick and thin.
4. through for now	4. I'm through for now.
5. go through	5. Go through here.
/hu/	
1. who knows	1. Who knows when?
2. who are	2. Who are you?
3. who will	3. I don't know who will.
4. who came	4. Who came last night?
5. who did	5. Who did you call?
/mju/	
1. sweet music	1. It's sweet music.
2. music makes	2. Music makes me happy.
3. all music	3. I like all music.
4. music hath	4. Music hath power _____.
5. music major	5. She's a music major.

/u/ CONTEXTS

Distinctive features: high-back, tense, round
/u/ ***consonant combinations:*** Final position of an unstressed syllable

Deep Test

/tu/ into

Common Words

/tu/
into

Everyday Language

Phrases

/tu/

1. go into
2. into it
3. get into
4. got into
5. into that

Sentences

1. Let's not go into that.
2. We're into it now.
3. We'll get into that next.
4. They got into it.
5. Into what–politics?

/ɝ/ CONTEXTS

Distinctive features: mid-central, tense, half-round, retroflexed (tongue tip up and back)
/ɝ/ ***consonant combinations:*** Initial position of a stressed syllable

Deep Test

/ɝ/ early   /ɝθ/ earth

Common Words

/ɝ/	/ɝθ/
early	earth

Everyday Language

Phrases	*Sentences*
/ɝ/	
1. you're early	1. You're early today.
2. early show	2. What's the early show?
3. get up early	3. We have to get up early.
4. early to bed	4. Early to bed, early to rise!
5. early bird	5. The early bird _____.
/ɝθ/	
1. on earth	1. What on earth is that?
2. heaven and earth	2. We're between heaven and earth.
3. is the earth	3. How big is the earth?
4. earth turns	4. The earth turns once how often?
5. smell the earth	5. Can you smell the earth?

/ɝ/ CONTEXTS

Distinctive features: mid-central, tense, half-round, retroflexed (tongue tip up and back)

/ɝ/ consonant combinations: Medial position of a stressed syllable

Deep Test

/wɝ/ word	/tɝ/ turn	/fɝ/ first	/sɝ/ serve	/lɝ/ learn
/bɝ/ bird	/hɝ/ hurt	/gɝ/ girl	/θɝ/ third	/tʃɝ/ church

Common Words

/wɝ/	/bɝ/	/tɝ/	/hɝ/	/fɝ/	/gɝ/	/sɝ/	/θɝ/
word	bird	return	heard	first	girl	serve	third
work	burn	turn	hurt				
world							
worth							

/lɝ/	/tʃɝ/
learn	church

Everyday Language

Phrases	*Sentences*
/wɝ/	
1. good word	1. What's the good word?
2. got to work	2. I got to work late.
3. in the world	3. Where in the world are you?
4. one word	4. One word and I'll poke him.
5. get to work	5. Let's get to work.
/bɝ/	
1. the red bird	1. Look at the red bird!
2. a bad burn	2. Was it a bad burn?
3. a bird dog	3. He has a bird dog.
4. burn everything	4. They burn everything!
5. burn the toast	5. Did you burn the toast?
/tɝ/	
1. the return address	1. What's the return address?
2. return it	2. You can return it.
3. turn around	3. Turn around slowly.
4. turn off	4. Turn off here and stop.
5. return soon	5. We'll have to return soon.
/hɝ/	
1. I heard	1. I heard about it.
2. hurt a little	2. It'll only hurt a little.
3. don't hurt me	3. Don't hurt me, please.
4. have you heard	4. Have you heard that song?
5. feelings were hurt	5. Her feelings were hurt.
/fɝ/	
1. here first	1. We were here first.
2. first we work	2. First we work, then play.
3. first place	3. Who won first place?
4. first time	4. The first time it was fun.
5. first things	5. First things first!
/gɝ/	
1. the new girl	1. Who's the new girl?
2. my girl	2. My girl called me.
3. is that girl	3. Is that girl here today?
4. girl crazy	4. He's kind of "girl crazy."
5. there's one girl	5. There's one girl too many.

Phrases	*Sentences*
/sɝ/	
1. do they serve	1. What kind do they serve?
2. serve yourself	2. Serve yourself, please.
3. your serve	3. It's your serve.
4. my third serve	4. This is my third serve.
5. serve food	5. Do they serve food here?
/θɝ/	
1. the third out	1. That's the third out.
2. you're third	2. You're third on the list.
3. third place	3. Third place went to Bill.
4. to be third	4. We're lucky to be third.
5. a third chance	5. Give me a third chance.
/lɝ/	
1. learn tomorrow	1. I'll learn tomorrow.
2. every learn	2. Won't they ever learn?
3. learn your lesson	3. Learn your lesson well.
4. learn quickly	4. He will learn quickly.
5. learn to learn	5. Learn to learn is a good rule.
/tʃɝ/	
1. the church supper	1. When is the church supper?
2. church was out	2. Church was out early.
3. at the church	3. They'll meet at the church.
4. church bells	4. Church bells sound nice.
5. a church mouse	5. He's poor as a church mouse.

/ɝ/ CONTEXTS

Distinctive features: mid-central, tense, half-round, retroflexed (tongue tip up and back)

/ɝ/ ***consonant combinations:*** Final position of a stressed syllable

Deep Test

/sɝ/ certain   /dʒɝ/ journal   /θɝ/ thirty   /hɝ/ hurry   /wɝ/ were
/pɝ/ purpose   /fɝ/ further

Common Words

/sɝ/	/pɝ/	/dʒɝ/	/fɝ/	/θɝ/	/hɝ/	/wɝ/
certain	person	journal	further	thirty	hurry	were
certainly	purpose					
service						
sir						

Everyday Language

Phrases	*Sentences*
/sɝ/	
1. certain of that	1. Are you certain of that?
2. certainly hope so	2. I certainly hope so.
3. quick service	3. That's quick service.
4. help you sir	4. May I help you, sir?
5. certain to win	5. We're certain to win now.
/pɝ/	
1. one person	1. One person at a time, please.
2. what's the purpose	2. What's the purpose of that?
3. no real purpose	3. I see no real purpose.
4. a good person	4. She's a good person.
5. my purpose	5. My purpose is to help.
/dʒɝ/	
1. that journal	1. That journal is old.
2. journal articles	2. Journal articles are dull.
3. new journal	3. This is a new journal.
4. read the journal	4. Did you read the journal?
5. the journal	5. The journal accepted my paper.
/fɝ/	
1. further your cause	1. We can't further your cause.
2. further in debt	2. Now we're even further in debt.
3. furthermore	3. Furthermore, I quit today!
4. further directions	4. Are there any further directions?
5. any further nominations	5. Are there any further nominations?
/θɝ/	
1. thirty days	1. Thirty days hath September . . .
2. thirty degrees	2. It's about thirty degrees.
3. thirty days	3. It's due in thirty days.
4. thirty minutes	4. She'll be here in thirty minutes.
5. thirty-year	5. They have a thirty-year lease.

Phrases	*Sentences*
/hɝ/	
1. hurry on	1. Hurry on down!
2. your hurry	2. What's your hurry?
3. better hurry	3. You'd better hurry!
4. can't hurry	4. I can't hurry any faster.
5. need to hurry	5. There's no need to hurry.
/wɝ/	
1. were you	1. Where were you?
2. you were	2. If you were me, what would you do?
3. they were	3. They were really surprised.
4. we were	4. We were going to tell you.
5. some were	5. Some were later than usual.

/ɚ/ CONTEXTS

Distinctive features: mid-central, lax, unround to half-round, retroflexed
/ɚ/***consonant combinations:*** Medial position of an unstressed syllable

Deep Test

/wɚ/ forward /dɚ/ modern /kɚ/ record /fɚ/ effort /vɚ/ government

Common Words

/wɚ/	/dɚ/	/kɚ/	/fɚ/	/vɚ/
forward	modern	record	effort	government

Everyday Language

Phrases	*Sentences*
/wɚ/	
1. forward thinking	1. He's forward thinking.
2. too forward	2. She's too forward.
3. face forward	3. Face forward now.
4. forward motion	4. They called a penalty for forward motion.
5. in forward	5. Put it in forward.

Phrases	*Sentences*
/dɚ/	
1. modern looking	1. It's rather modern looking.
2. modern dance	2. Do you like modern dance?
3. modern look	3. This is the modern look.
4. little more modern	4. I'd like it a little more modern.
5. modern facilities	5. There are modern facilities there.
/kɚ/	
1. hear the record	1. Let's hear the record.
2. a hit record	2. They made a hit record.
3. this record	3. This record is scratchy.
4. your record	4. Who took your record?
5. my record	5. Put my record on top.
/fɚ/	
1. a little effort	1. Put out a little effort.
2. much effort	2. It doesn't take much effort.
3. your effort	3. Your effort is appreciated.
4. combined effort	4. With combined effort, we can.
5. appreciate the effort	5. You don't appreciate the effort.
/vɚ/	
1. government man	1. He's a government man.
2. government job	2. It's a government job.
3. federal government	3. The federal government owns it.
4. good government	4. Good government is hard to get.
5. student government	5. Are you in student government?

/ɚ/ CONTEXTS

Distinctive features: mid-central, lax, unround to half-round, retroflexed
/ɚ/ consonant combinations: Final position of an unstressed syllable

Deep Test

/tɚ/ after	/bɚ/ labor	/sɚ/ answer	/hɚ/ herself
/ðɚ/ other	/fɚ/ offer	/mɚ/ summer	/jɚ/ figure
/vɚ/ cover	/nɚ/ dinner	/dʒɚ/ danger	/ŋɚ/ finger
/dɚ/ order	/tʃɚ/ teacher	/ʒɚ/ measure	/wɚ/ flower
/pɚ/ paper	/gɚ/ sugar	/lɚ/ color	

Common Words

/tɚ/	/ðɚ/	/vɚ/	/dɚ/	/pɚ/
after	another	cover	consider	newspaper
afternoon	brother	discover	leader	paper
butter	either	ever	order	perhaps
center	father	favor	shoulder	permit
character	gather	however	under	proper
daughter	mother	never	understand	
doctor	neither	over	wonder	
enter	other	river	wonderful	
letter	rather	silver		
master	together	whatever		
matter	weather			
quarter	whether			
sister				
water				
winter				

/bɚ/	/nɚ/	/tʃɚ/	/sɚ/	/wɚ/	/fɚ/
labor	corner	future	answer	flower	forget
member	dinner	nature	exercise	lower	offer
neighbor	honor	picture	officer	power	suffer
number	manner	teacher			
remember					

/mɚ/	/dʒɚ/	/ʒɚ/	/lɚ/	/gɚ/	/hɚ/
farmer	danger	measure	color	finger	herself
summer	soldier	pleasure	dollar	sugar	

/jɚ/
figure

Everyday Language

Phrases	*Sentences*
/tɚ/	
1. letter here	1. There's a letter here for you.
2. some water	2. May I have some water?
3. what a winter	3. What a winter this is!
4. pass the butter	4. Please pass the butter.
5. after me	5. You're after me.

Phrases	*Sentences*
/ðɚ/	
1. neither one	1. Neither one will do.
2. crazy weather	2. This is crazy weather.
3. go together	3. Let's go together.
4. either you can	4. Either you can or you can't.
5. rather not	5. I'd rather not say.
/vɚ/	
1. a favor	1. Do me a favor?
2. ever end	2. Will it ever end?
3. cover on it	3. Just put a cover on it.
4. come over	4. Come over some time.
5. never make	5. I'll never make it!
/dɚ/	
1. your order	1. Is this your order?
2. I wonder	2. I wonder what happened?
3. you understand	3. You understand, don't you?
4. be the leader	4. You be the leader.
5. consider him	5. Did you consider him?
/pɚ/	
1. perhaps we	1. Perhaps we will.
2. permit it	2. They'll never permit it.
3. be proper	3. Would that be proper?
4. some paper	4. You'll need some paper.
5. seen the newspaper	5. Have you seen the newspaper?
/bɚ/	
1. your number	1. Your number is up.
2. remember it	2. Can you remember it?
3. your neighbor	3. Your neighbor came over.
4. in labor	4. She's in labor now.
5. I remember	5. I remember that all too well.
/nɚ/	
1. come for dinner	1. Can you come for dinner?
2. dark corner	2. This is such a dark corner.
3. pleasant manner	3. She has a pleasant manner.
4. your honor	4. Well, your honor, it's like this.
5. dinner is	5. Dinner is getting cold.

Phrases	*Sentences*
/tʃɚ/	
1. much future	1. There's not much future.
2. your teacher	2. Who's your teacher?
3. usual nature	3. It's not his usual nature.
4. picture of that	4. I have a picture of that!
5. nature study	5. We're taking nature study.
/sɚ/	
1. answer soon	1. We'll need your answer soon.
2. good exercise	2. That's good exercise.
3. an officer	3. He's an officer.
4. right answer	4. What's the right answer.
5. speeding officer	5. I wasn't speeding, Officer.
/wɚ/	
1. lower bunk	1. You get the lower bunk.
2. more power	2. More power to you!
3. send flowers	3. Let's send flowers.
4. lower the window	4. Lower the window a little.
5. the power	5. The power is off.
/fɚ/	
1. an offer	1. Make an offer.
2. needn't suffer	2. You needn't suffer.
3. your offer	3. Your offer is accepted.
4. offer still	4. Does your offer still hold?
5. just suffer	5. Just suffer in silence!
/mɚ/	
1. next summer	1. Next summer will be better.
2. be a farmer	2. Would you be a farmer?
3. being a farmer	3. It isn't easy being a farmer.
4. summer time	4. Summer time is great!
5. summer suit	5. Wear your summer suit.
/dʒɚ/	
1. little danger	1. There's little danger here.
2. soldier now	2. He's a soldier now.
3. danger sign	3. Did you see the danger sign?
4. danger was	4. Danger was everywhere!
5. that soldier	5. Let's ask that soldier.

Phrases	*Sentences*
/ʒɚ/	
1. measure it	1. We'd better measure it.
2. measure up	2. It doesn't measure up.
3. your pleasure	3. What's your pleasure?
4. pleasure trip	4. This is a pleasure trip.
5. full measure	5. They give you full measure.
/lɚ/	
1. a dollar	1. Here's a dollar.
2. color it	2. Color it "happy"!
3. your color	3. Your color is good.
4. a dollar should	4. A dollar should do it.
5. my dollar	5. Here's my dollar.
/gɚ/	
1. the sugar	1. Pass the sugar, please.
2. your finger	2. Put your finger in it.
3. needs sugar	3. It needs sugar.
4. sugar is sweet	4. Sugar is sweet and _____.
5. one finger	5. Hold up one finger.
/hɚ/	
1. caused it herself	1. She caused it herself.
2. blame herself	2. She can blame herself.
3. thank herself	3. She should thank herself.
4. consider herself	4. She should consider herself lucky.
5. for herself	5. She kept it for herself.
/jɚ/	
1. nice figure	1. She has a nice figure.
2. I figure	2. I figure it will work out.
3. figure that	3. How do you figure that?
4. figure it	4. Did they figure it right?
5. lowest figure	5. Is that the lowest figure?
/ŋɚ/	

/ʌ/ CONTEXTS

Distinctive features: low-back-central, lax, unround
/ʌ/ ***consonant combinations:*** Initial position of a stressed syllable

Deep Test

/ʌp/ up   /ʌð/ other   /ʌs/ us   /ʌn/ under   /ʌŋ/ uncle

Common Words

/ʌp/	/ʌð/	/ʌs/	/ʌn/	/ʌŋ/
up	other	us	under	uncle

Everyday Language

Phrases	*Sentences*
/ʌp/	
1. on up	1. Come on up!
2. up up	2. Up, up, and away!
3. what's up	3. What's up now?
4. up or down	4. You're either up or down.
5. run up	5. Don't run up the bill.
/ʌð/	
1. the other	1. It's one or the other.
2. the other one	2. Where's the other one?
3. other shoe	3. I lost my other shoe.
4. without the other	4. What's one without the other?
5. other fellow	5. Who's the other fellow?
/ʌs/	
1. one of us	1. Now there's one of us.
2. us or them	2. It's us or them.
3. with us	3. Are you with us?
4. give us	4. Give us a chance.
5. give us more	5. Give us more time.
/ʌn/	
1. under you	1. Is he under you?
2. under pressure	2. He's under pressure now.
3. under the bed	3. Hide it under the bed.
4. under any circumstances	4. I won't under any circumstances.
5. stand under	5. Stand under the tree.

Phrases	*Sentences*
/ʌŋ/	
1. uncle sam	1. Uncle Sam wants you!
2. say uncle	2. Say "uncle" and I'll stop.
3. your uncle	3. Is he your uncle?
4. monkey's uncle	4. Well, I'll be a monkey's uncle!
5. have an uncle	5. I have an uncle named ____.

/ʌ/ CONTEXTS

Distinctive features: low-back-central, lax, unround
/ʌ/ ***consonant combinations:*** Medial position of a stressed syllable

Deep Test

/sʌ/ some	/bʌ/ above	/frʌ/ from	/zʌ/ result
/kʌ/ come	/dʒʌ/ just	/lʌ/ love	/jʌ/ young
/mʌ/ money	/hʌ/ hundred	/pʌ/ public	/blʌ/ blood
/nʌ/ nothing	/rʌ/ run	/tʌ/ touch	/klʌ/ club
/wʌ/ one	/trʌ/ trouble	/gʌ/ government	/stʌ/ study
/dʌ/ done			

Common Words

/sʌ/	/kʌ/	/mʌ/	/nʌ/	/wʌ/	/dʌ/
some	become	among	another	once	does
something	color	money	enough	one	doesn't
sometimes	come	month	none	was	done
son	coming	mother	nothing	wonder	double
subject	company	much	number	wonderful	
such	country	must			
sudden	cover				
suddenly	cup				
suffer	discover				
summer					
sun					

/bʌ/	/dʒʌ/	/hʌ/	/rʌ/	/trʌ/	/frʌ/	/lʌ/	/pʌ/
above	judge	hundred	run	trouble	from	love	public
but	just	husband	rush	trust	front		
butter							

/tʌ/	/gʌ/	/zʌ/	/jʌ/	/blʌ/	/klʌ/	/stʌ/
touch	government	result	young	blood	club	study

Everyday Language

Phrases	*Sentences*
/sʌ/	
1. like some	1. Would you like some?
2. something tells	2. Something tells me no.
3. sometimes I'm	3. Sometimes I'm not sure.
4. suddenly it	4. Suddenly it was over!
5. summer is	5. Summer is fun.
/kʌ/	
1. become of it	1. What'll become of it?
2. favorite color	2. My favorite color is _____.
3. two's company	3. Two's company, three's _____.
4. I'm coming	4. Hold it, I'm coming!
5. cup of wine	5. Add a cup of wine to it.
/mʌ/	
1. money talks	1. Money talks, right?
2. among men	2. He's a giant among men.
3. my mother	3. My mother told me so.
4. how much	4. How much is it?
5. you must	5. You must believe me.
/nʌ/	
1. just another	1. It's just another day.
2. had enough	2. Had enough now?
3. none left	3. There's none left.
4. nothing more	4. I've nothing more to say.
5. your number	5. Your number is up.
/wʌ/	
1. went once	1. I went once.
2. one time	2. One time is enough.
3. was here	3. He was here today.
4. I wonder	4. I wonder what happened.
5. was wonderful	5. It was wonderful!
/dʌ/	
1. does it say	1. What does it say?
2. doesn't make	2. It doesn't make sense.
3. done it	3. Now you done it.
4. double or nothing	4. Double or nothing, OK?
5. does it do	5. What good does it do?

Phrases	*Sentences*
/bʌ/	
1. above all	1. Above all, don't stop.
2. but when	2. We'll go, but when?
3. butter and toast	3. I love butter and toast.
4. above you	4. Look above you.
5. but you	5. They're all here but you.
/dʒʌ/	
1. just know it	1. You just know it!
2. be the judge	2. You be the judge.
3. I suggest	3. I suggest you stop.
4. just now	4. Just now I can't.
5. do you suggest	5. What do you suggest?
/hʌ/	
1. bet a hundred	1. I'll bet a hundred.
2. husband do	2. What does your husband do?
3. hundred to one	3. It's a hundred to one.
4. husband works	4. My husband works.
5. husband come	5. Did your husband come?
/rʌ/	
1. rush me	1. Don't rush me!
2. I'll run	2. I'll run if you can't.
3. who'll run	3. Who'll run for secretary?
4. rush please	4. Mark it RUSH, please.
5. rush out	5. Rush out and buy one!
/trʌ/	
1. trouble is	1. The trouble is, I'm broke.
2. don't trust	2. I don't trust her.
3. trouble now	3. What's the trouble now?
4. trust me	4. You can trust me.
5. much trouble	5. It's too much trouble.
/frʌ/	
1. from here	1. It's too far from here.
2. the front	2. Face the front.
3. in front	3. Put it in front.
4. from there	4. Take it from there.
5. from here	5. From here to there is an hour.

Phrases	*Sentences*
/lʌ/	
1. love it	1. I love it!
2. love you	2. She'll love you.
3. love is	3. Love is blind.
4. love was	4. Love was everywhere.
5. all love	5. We all love you.
/pʌ/	
1. make it public	1. Why make it public?
2. public figure	2. He's a public figure.
3. public knows	3. The public knows.
4. public knowledge	4. It's public knowledge.
5. public support	5. Public support helps.
/tʌ/	
1. the touch	1. It's the touch of genius.
2. you touch	2. You touch me.
3. touch me	3. Touch me and I'll scream!
4. Midas touch	4. He has the "Midas touch."
5. touch it	5. Touch it lightly.
/gʌ/	
1. local government	1. Local government should solve it.
2. state government	2. State government can help out.
3. federal government	3. Finally, there's the federal government.
4. world government	4. What about world government?
5. big government	5. That's a big government!
/zʌ/	
1. the result	1. What's the result?
2. result is	2. The result is good.
3. good result	3. One good result helps.
4. will result	4. It will result in victory.
5. that result	5. Do you promise that result?
/jʌ/	
1. young once	1. You're only young once.
2. feel young	2. I feel young.
3. look young	3. You look young.
4. am young	4. I am young!
5. young enough	5. Well, you're young enough.

Phrases	*Sentences*
/blʌ/	
1. his blood	1. It's in his blood.
2. much blood	2. Did he lose much blood?
3. blood is	3. Blood is thicker than water.
4. my blood	4. My blood ran cold!
5. blood relative	5. He's a blood relative.
/klʌ/	
1. the club	1. Join the club!
2. club meets	2. Tonight my club meets.
3. which club	3. Which club is that?
4. bridge club	4. It's my bridge club.
5. a club	5. A club can be fun.
/stʌ/	
1. to study	1. I have to study.
2. you study	2. What will you study?
3. study history	3. I need to study history.
4. lot of study	4. That takes a lot of study.
5. my study	5. Come into my study.

/ə/ CONTEXTS

Distinctive features: low-mid-central, lax, unround to half-round
/ə/ ***consonant combinations:*** Initial position of an unstressed syllable

Deep Test

/ə/ about	/əd/ method	/əb/ obtain	/ənd/ second
/ən/ given	/əl/ material	/əs/ various	/əns/ experience

Common Words

/ə/	/ən/	/əl/	/əb/	/əd/	/əs/
about	broken	general	obtain	method	various
above	common	material	object	period	
according	condition	national	probably		
account	given	real			
across	happen	realize			
affair	heaven	special			
afraid	often				
again	position				
against	seven				
ago	taken				
agree	unless				
allow	until				
alone	woman				
along					
among					
amount					
another					
appear					
around					
arrive					
attempt					
attention					
away					
opinion					
upon					

/ənd/	/əns/
second	experience

Everyday Language

Phrases	*Sentences*
/ə/	
1. about time	1. It's about time.
2. according to this	2. According to this, you're late.
3. afraid so	3. I'm afraid so.
4. you agree	4. Do you agree?
5. come along	5. We've come along quickly.

Phrases	*Sentences*
/ən/	
1. common cold	1. The common cold is bad.
2. given up	2. He's about given up.
3. happen now	3. What'll happen now?
4. taken all	4. I've taken all I can.
5. happen often	5. It doesn't happen often.
/əl/	
1. general statement	1. That's a general statement.
2. realize it	2. Do you realize it?
3. real tiger	3. She's a real tiger!
4. what's special	4. What's special about it?
5. national bank	5. Where's the National Bank?
/əb/	
1. I object	1. I object, your honor!
2. you object	2. Why do you object?
3. probably doesn't	3. He probably doesn't know.
4. you obtain	4. Can you obtain an extra one?
5. probably not	5. Probably not now.
/əd/	
1. new method	1. There's a new method.
2. slow period	2. This is a slow period.
3. what method	3. What method do you use?
4. put a period	4. Put a period after it.
5. first period	5. First period is math.
/əs/	
1. various ways	1. There are various ways.
2. various people	2. Various people come here.
3. are various	3. Weather conditions are various now
4. various reasons	4. For various reasons, we can't.
5. various opinions	5. There are various opinions.
/ənd/	
1. second best	1. It's second best.
2. came in second	2. You came in second.
3. second or third	3. Second or third is OK!
4. second rate	4. The movie is second rate.
5. second guess	5. Don't second guess me.

Phrases	*Sentences*
/əns/	
1. good experience	1. It'll be good experience.
2. bad experience	2. Last time was a bad experience.
3. experience always	3. Experience always helps.
4. need experience	4. You'll need experience.
5. your experience	5. Where did you get your experience?

/ə/ CONTEXTS

Distinctive features: low-mid-central, lax, unround to half-round
/ə/ ***consonant combinations:*** Medial position of an unstressed syllable

Deep Test

/mə/ famous	/lə/ island	/fə/ beautiful	/bə/ husband
/kə/ complete	/tə/ distance	/sə/ supply	/və/ even
/ʃə/ action	/də/ industry	/rə/ several	/ðə/ themselves
/jə/ million	/pə/ open	/drə/ children	/tʃə/ mention

COMMON WORDS

/mə/	/kə/	/ʃə/	/jə/	/lə/	/tə/
department	complete	action	million	island	distance
famous	condition	attention	opinion	problem	system
gentleman	consider	direction	question	silence	
government	contain	nation	union		
human	continue	ocean			
moment	control	station			
movement					

/də/	/pə/	/fə/	/sə/	/rə/	/drə/
industry	open	beautiful	success	natural	children
president	purpose	wonderful	supply	several	

/bə/	/və/	/ðə/	/tʃə/
husband	even	themselves	mention

Everyday Language

Phrases	*Sentences*
/mə/	
1. shoe department	1. Where's the shoe department?
2. famous person	2. He's a famous person.
3. be a gentleman	3. Always be a gentleman.
4. only human	4. We're only human.
5. a moment	5. Wait a moment.
/kə/	
1. it's complete	1. Now it's complete.
2. one conditon	2. I will on one condition.
3. continue tomorrow	3. Let's continue tomorrow.
4. lost control	4. I think we've lost control.
5. consider the source	5. Just consider the source.
/ʃə/	
1. some action	1. Let's have some action!
2. attention everyone	2. Attention, everyone, attention!
3 which direction	3. Which direction now?
4. one nation	4. "One nation, indivisible . . ."
5. next station	5. Stop at the next station.
/jə/	
1. in a million	1. It's one chance in a million.
2. your opinion	2. That's your opinion.
3. the question	3. What's the question?
4. join the union	4. Did you join the union?
5. a million dollars	5. Not for a million dollars!
/lə/	
1. an island	1. No man is an island.
2. the problem	2. That's the problem.
3. silence is	3. Silence is golden.
4. your problem	4. What's your problem?
5. silence is awful	5. The silence is awful.
/tə/	
1. quite a distance	1. It's quite a distance.
2. the system	2. You can't beat the system.
3. distance runner	3. He's a distance runner.
4. long distance	4. Call long distance.
5. new system	5. How's the new system.

Phrases	*Sentences*
/də/	
1. for president	1. He'll run for president.
2. president is	2. President _____ is in the White House.
3. what industry	3. What industry makes clothing?
4. industry helps	4. Industry helps cities.
5. be president	5. Would you be president?
/pə/	
1. open book	1. It's an open book.
2. what purpose	2. What purpose will it serve?
3. open up	3. Open up now.
4. the purpose	4. The purpose is clear.
5. on purpose	5. You did that on purpose!
/fə/	
1. beautiful day	1. What a beautiful day!
2. is wonderful	2. Life is wonderful!
3. beautiful lady	3. She's a beautiful lady.
4. it's wonderful	4. It's wonderful to be here.
5. wonderful fool	5. You're a wonderful fool!
/sə/	
1. a success	1. Now you're a success.
2. success takes	2. Success takes work.
3. short supply	3. That's in short supply.
4. you supply	4. You supply the brains!
5. beat success	5. You can't beat success.
/rə/	
1. just natural	1. It's just natural.
2. several times	2. He came several times.
3. natural thing	3. Its the natural thing to do.
4. several books	4. He has several books.
5. natural food	5. Natural food is best.
/drə/	
1. children pay	1. Children, pay attention!
2. like children	2. Do you like children?
3. act like children	3. They act like children.
4. for children	4. Christmas is for children.
5. for the children	5. Watch out for the children!

Phrases	*Sentences*
/bə/	
1. your husband	1. Do I know your husband?
2. give your husband	2. What did you give your husband.
3. my husband	3. My husband won't go.
4. her husband	4. Her husband told me.
5. husband stealer	5. She's a husband stealer!
/və/	
1. we're even	1. Now we're even.
2. even now	2. Even now I'm scared!
3. even speak	3. She wouldn't even speak.
4. even lengths	4. Make them even lengths.
5. even fit me	5. That'll even fit me!
/ðə/	
1. do it themselves	1. They can do it themselves.
2. for themselves	2. It's just for themselves.
3. can't see themselves	3. People can't see themselves.
4. hear themselves	4. If they could only hear themselves.
5. help themselves	5. They should help themselves.
/tʃə/	
1. mention it	1. Don't mention it.
2. mention my name	2. Just mention my name.
3. didn't mention	3. They didn't mention going.
4. mention it	4. Mention it to him.
5. honorable mention	5. That's honorable mention.

/ə/ CONTEXTS

Distinctive features: low-mid-central, lax, unround to half-round
/ə/ ***consonant combinations:*** Final position of an unstressed syllable

Deep Test

/sə/ society	/tə/ today	/pə/ position	/prə/ provide	/tʃə/ century
/bə/ believe	/də/ direct	/mə/ machine	/kə/ command	

Common Words

/sə/	/bə/	/tə/	/də/	/pə/	/mə/
society	believe	beautiful	direct	company	machine
support	belong	today	direction	position	material
suppose	below	together	divide		
surprise	between	tomorrow			
necessary					
possible					

/prə/	/kə/	/tʃə/
produce	command	century
provide		

Everyday Language

Phrases	*Sentences*
/sə/	
1. high society	1. We're in high society!
2. do you suppose	2. Do you suppose we are?
3. surprise you	3. It would surprise you.
4. need support	4. We'll need support.
5. suppose so	5. I suppose so.
/bə/	
1. believe it	1. You better believe it.
2. does it belong	2. Where does it belong?
3. down below	3. Put it down below.
4. between us	4. Sit between us.
5. below her	5. You're below her.
/tə/	
1. today we can	1. Today we can start.
2. go together	2. Let's go together.
3. tomorrow will be	3. Tomorrow will be better.
4. beautiful story	4. It's a beautiful story.
5. after today	5. After today, we'll know.

Phrases	*Sentences*
/də/	
1. be direct	1. Be direct now!
2. need direction	2. We'll need direction.
3. divide it	3. Divide it up.
4. direct quote	4. That's a direct quote.
5. which direction	5. Which direction is it?
/pə/	
1. two's company	1. Two's company, _____.
2. sitting position	2. Take a sitting position.
3. new position	3. It's a new position.
4. some company	4. Want some company?
5. company policy	5. That's company policy.
/mə/	
1. the machine	1. Fix the machine.
2. new material	2. We need new material.
3. material wrinkles	3. That material wrinkles.
4. new machine	4. We're getting a new machine.
5. machine age	5. This is the machine age.
/prə/	
1. provide the money	1. They'll provide the money.
2. produce it	2. We can produce it here.
3. produce new ideas	3. It'll produce new ideas.
4. provide the paper	4. Will you provide the paper?
5. will provide	5. Nature will provide.
/kə/	
1. command you	1. I command you!
2. the command	2. Give the command.
3. in command	3. Who'll be in command?
4. to command	4. There's no one to command.
5. command attention	5. It'll certainly command attention.
/tʃə/	
1. century ago	1. It was a century ago.
2. a century	2. A century is _____ years.
3. eighteenth century	3. This is eighteenth century music.
4. this century	4. Who was the greatest woman of this century?
5. twentieth century	5. It reads like the twentieth century.

DIPHTHONGS

/aɪ/ CONTEXTS

Distinctive features: glide combination from /a/ to /ɪ/
/aɪ/ ***consonant combinations:*** Initial position of a stressed syllable

Deep Test

/aɪ/ eye /aɪd/ I'd /aɪs/ ice /aɪm/ I'm /aɪl/ I'll

Common Words

/aɪ/	/aɪd/	/aɪs/	/aɪm/	/aɪl/
eye	I'd	ice	I'm	I'll
I				
iron				
island				

Everyday Language

Phrases	***Sentences***
/aɪ/	
1. eye open	1. Keep an eye open.
2. I will	2. I will if you will.
3. made of iron	3. He's made of iron.
4. an island	4. No man is an island.
5. in the eye	5. Look me in the eye.
/aɪd/	
1. I'd rather	1. I'd rather not go.
2. I'd tell you	2. I'd tell you if I could.
3. I'd seen	3. He asked if I'd seen you.
4. I'd finished	4. He came after I'd finished.
5. I'd started	5. I'd started already.

Phrases	*Sentences*
/aɪs/	
1. cold as ice	1. It's cold as ice.
2. ice cream	2. I love ice cream.
3. snow and ice	3. They're predicting snow and ice.
4. ice cubes	4. Ice cubes are handy.
5. ice the cake	5. Ice the cake later.
/aɪm/	
1. I'm tired	1. I'm tired of this.
2. I'm going	2. I'm going home.
3. where I'm going	3. I don't know where I'm going.
4. I'm not	4. I'm not ready.
5. I'm your	5. I'm your friend.
/aɪl/	
1. I'll tell	1. I'll tell you later.
2. I'll know	2. I'll know more tomorrow.
3. I'll help	3. You bet I'll help!
4. I'll go	4. I'll go if you will.
5. I'll be	5. I'll be darned!

/aɪ/ CONTEXTS

Distinctive features: glide combination from /a/ to /ɪ/
/aɪ/ ***consonant combinations:*** Initial position of an unstressed syllable

Deep Test

/aɪ/ idea

Common Words

/aɪ/
idea

Everyday Language

Phrases	*Sentences*
/aɪ/	
1. good idea	1. That's a good idea.
2. that idea	2. That idea is popular.
3. whose idea	3. Whose idea is this?
4. one idea	4. One idea is best.
5. this idea	5. Who gave you this idea?

/aɪ/ CONTEXTS

Distinctive features: glide combination from /a/ to /ɪ/
/aɪ/ ***consonant combinations:*** Medial position of a stressed syllable

Deep Test

/saɪ/ beside	/naɪ/ night	/praɪ/ price	/tʃaɪ/ child
/faɪ/ five	/taɪ/ time	/kwaɪ/ require	/traɪ/ tried
/raɪ/ arrive	/vaɪ/ divide	/kaɪ/ kind	/draɪ/ drive
/maɪ/ might	/haɪ/ height	/gaɪ/ guide	/smaɪ/ smile
/laɪ/ like	/hwaɪ/ white	/zaɪ/ desire	/braɪ/ bright
/waɪ/ wide			

Common Words

/saɪ/	/faɪ/	/raɪ/	/maɪ/	/laɪ/	/waɪ/	/naɪ/	/taɪ/
beside	fight	arrive	might	life	wide	night	time
decide	find	ride	mile	light	wife	nice	tire
outside	fine	right	mind	like	wild	nine	type
side	fire	rise	mine	line	wise		
sight	five	write					
sign							
size							

/vaɪ/	/haɪ/	/hwaɪ/	/praɪ/	/kwaɪ/	/kaɪ/	/gaɪ/
divide	behind	while	price	quiet	kind	guide
provide	height	white	surprise	require		

/zaɪ/	/tʃaɪ/	/traɪ/	/draɪ/	/smaɪ/	/braɪ/
desire	child	tried	drive	smile	bright

Everyday Language

Phrases	*Sentences*
/saɪ/	
1. beside myself	1. I'm just beside myself!
2. can't decide	2. He can't decide for you.
3. go outside	3. Let's go outside.
4. stop sign	4. Watch for the stop sign.
5. what size	5. What size do you take?
/faɪ/	
1. fight for	1. Fight for your rights!
2. find one	2. Where can I find one?
3. I'm fine	3. I'm fine, thanks.
4. fire you	4. They'll fire you if you go.
5. five times	5. What's five times five?
/raɪ/	
1. arrive late	1. They'll arrive late.
2. need a ride	2. Do you need a ride?
3. you're right	3. You're right, it's cold!
4. early to rise	4. Early to bed, early to rise . . .
5. write me	5. Write me a note, please.
/maɪ/	
1. might be	1. I might be able to go.
2. a mile	2. You missed by a mile!
3. won't mind	3. She won't mind.
4. use mine	4. You may use mine.
5. just might	5. I just might do that.
/laɪ/	
1. good life	1. It's a good life.
2. have a light	2. Do you have a light?
3. like it	3. Try it, you'll like it!
4. a line	4. Drop me a line sometime.
5. the light	5. Turn on the light.
/waɪ/	
1. wide berth	1. Give them a wide berth.
2. your wife	2. How's your wife?
3. little wild	3. Things are a little wild now.
4. think it's wise	4. Do you think it's wise?
5. wild ride	5. That was a wild ride!

Phrases	*Sentences*
/naɪ/	
1. night game	1. Is there a night game?
2. nice person	2. She's a nice person.
3. nine lives	3. A cat has nine lives, they say.
4. good night	4. Good night now.
5. nice time	5. It's been a nice time.
/taɪ/	
1. good time	1. Have a good time!
2. flat tire	2. You have a flat tire.
3. what type	3. What type does it take?
4. more time	4. I need more time.
5. my type	5. She's not my type.
/vaɪ/	
1. we'll divide	1. We'll divide the spoils!
2. provide the drinks	2. Can you provide the drinks?
3. divide it	3. Divide it up evenly.
4. provide assistance	4. They provide assistance.
5. divide and conquer	5. "Divide and conquer," they say.
/haɪ/	
1. what's behind	1. What's behind that wall?
2. height makes	2. Height makes a difference.
3. new heights	3. He soared to new heights.
4. far behind	4. I'm so far behind!
5. way behind	5. We're all way behind.
/hwaɪ/	
1. while you're gone	1. While you're gone, I'll do it.
2. black or white	2. It's either black or white.
3. while we eat	3. Let's rest while we eat.
4. while I'm gone	4. While I'm gone, do it.
5. white one	5. Take the white one.
/praɪ/	
1. price is	1. The price is good.
2. have a surprise	2. I have a surprise for you.
3. good price	3. What's a good price?
4. that's a surprise	4. That's a surprise to me.
5. regular price	5. It's half of the regular price.

Phrases	*Sentences*
/kwaɪ/	
1. quiet evening	1. We had a quiet evening.
2. require a license	2. That will require a license.
3. be quiet	3. Let's be quiet.
4. quiet down	4. Quiet down, everybody!
5. require experience	5. We don't require experience.
/kaɪ/	
1. be kind	1. Be kind to him.
2. what kind	2. What kind do you like?
3. this kind	3. This kind is old fashioned.
4. his kind	4. His kind never help.
5. any kind	5. Any kind will do.
/gaɪ/	
1. hire a guide	1. We'll hire a guide.
2. tour guide	2. Let's ask the tour guide.
3. guide you	3. The signs will guide you.
4. guide to	4. Guide to the right now.
5. guide on	5. Guide on, I'll follow.
/zaɪ/	
1. one desire	1. I have one desire.
2. do you desire	2. What do you desire?
3. my desire	3. My desire is small.
4. any desire	4. Any desire is hard to get.
5. my desire is	5. My desire is to be rich!
/tʃaɪ/	
1. your child	1. Is this your child?
2. like a child	2. She acts like a child.
3. even a child	3. Even a child can do it.
4. my child	4. Patience, my child!
5. one child	5. One child is enough.
/traɪ/	
1. tried everything	1. I've tried everything!
2. tried aspirin	2. Have you tried aspirin?
3. they tried	3. They tried to call you.
4. we tried	4. We tried and tried, but lost.
5. tried and true	5. She's a tried and true friend.

Phrases	*Sentences*
/draɪ/	
1. drive today	1. Can you drive today?
2. a lot of drive	2. He has a lot of drive.
3. drive me	3. They drive me crazy!
4. drive on	4. Drive on, my friend!
5. short drive	5. It's just a short drive.
/smaɪ/	
1. smile awhile	1. Smile awhile, it's alright.
2. pretty smile	2. She has a pretty smile.
3. makes me smile	3. Sunshine makes me smile.
4. smile a day	4. Try a smile a day.
5. smile when	5. Smile when you say that, pahdnuh!
/braɪ/	
1. really bright	1. He's really bright.
2. bright light	2. That's sure a bright light!
3. bright idea	3. I have a bright idea!
4. too bright	4. The sun is too bright now.
5. star bright	5. Star light, star bright . . .

/aɪ/ CONTEXTS

Distinctive features: glide combination from /a/ to /ɪ/
/aɪ/ ***consonant combinations:*** Medial position of an unstressed syllable

Deep Test

/taɪ/ sometimes /saɪ/ exercise /laɪ/ realize

Common Words

/taɪ/	/saɪ/	/laɪ/
sometimes	exercise	realize

Everyday Language

Phrases	*Sentences*
/taɪ/	
1. sometimes I'm	1. Sometimes I'm happy.
2. together sometimes	2. Let's go together sometimes.
3. angry sometimes	3. You make me angry sometimes.
4. sometimes it's	4. Sometimes it's too late.
5. sometimes it pays	5. Sometimes it pays to wait.
/saɪ/	
1. good exercise	1. That's good exercise.
2. exercise is	2. Exercise is good for you.
3. wasted exercise	3. It's a wasted exercise.
4. first exercise	4. Do the first exercise.
5. will exercise	5. It will exercise your mind.
/laɪ/	
1. didn't realize	1. I didn't realize.
2. you realize	2. Do you realize what's happening?
3. realize it	3. They realize it now.
4. you'll realize	4. You'll realize a savings.
5. I realize	5. I realize you can't.

/aɪ/ CONTEXTS

Distinctive features: glide combination from /a/ to /ɪ/
/aɪ/ ***consonant combinations:*** Final position of a stressed syllable

Deep Test

/baɪ/ by	/daɪ/ die	/laɪ/ lie	/kraɪ/ cry
/saɪ/ silence	/faɪ/ finally	/hwaɪ/ why	/flaɪ/ fly
/plaɪ/ reply	/haɪ/ high	/traɪ/ try	/skaɪ/ sky
/taɪ/ tie	/maɪ/ my	/draɪ/ dry	

Common Words

/baɪ/	/saɪ/	/plaɪ/	/taɪ/	/daɪ/	/faɪ/	/haɪ/	/maɪ/
buy	silence	reply	tie	die	finally	high	my
by	society	supply					

/laɪ/	/hwaɪ/	/traɪ/	/draɪ/	/kraɪ/	/flaɪ/	/skaɪ/
lie	why	try	dry	cry	fly	sky

Everyday Language

Phrases	*Sentences*
/baɪ/	
1. buy that	1. Where did you buy that?
2. by me	2. Sit by me, OK?
3. don't buy	3. I don't buy that line.
4. by myself	4. I can do it by myself.
5. buy me	5. Buy me a coke, please?
/saɪ/	
1. silence is golden	1. Silence is golden, they say.
2. high society	2. We're in high society.
3. our society	3. Our society doesn't allow it.
4. the silence	4. The silence scares me.
5. silence please	5. Silence please, we're starting.
/plaɪ/	
1. the reply	1. What's the reply?
2. good supply	2. That's in good supply.
3. my reply	3. My reply is _____.
4. our supply	4. Our supply is gone.
5. supply and demand	5. Supply and demand is the key.
/taɪ/	
1. nice tie	1. That's a nice tie.
2. tie it	2. Tie it tight.
3. can you tie	3. Can you tie a square knot?
4. in a tie	4. It ended in a tie.
5. tie games	5. Tie games are exciting!

Phrases	*Sentences*
/daɪ/	
1. may die	1. I think I may die!
2. do or die	2. "Do or die" is their motto.
3. won't die	3. You won't die from work.
4. they'll die	4. They'll die like flies.
5. die sometime	5. We all have to die sometime.
/faɪ/	
1. finally happened	1. It finally happened.
2. finally it's	2. Finally it's finished.
3. today finally	3. We'll know today, finally.
4. finally came	4. It finally came.
5. finally told us	5. He finally told us.
/haɪ/	
1. high old time	1. We had a high old time!
2. too high	2. The price is too high.
3. high time	3. It's high time!
4. high hopes	4. We have high hopes.
5. high today	5. The high today was 80°.
/maɪ/	
1. my time	1. My time is limited.
2. my job	2. I know my job.
3. my turn	3. When my turn comes I'm ready.
4. my share	4. Put my share in.
5. my place	5. My place is with you.
/laɪ/	
1. lie down	1. Lie down and rest.
2. don't lie	2. Don't lie to me!
3. big lie	3. That's a big lie!
4. we lie	4. Where should we lie?
5. lie close	5. Lie close to me.
/hwaɪ/	
1. why can't	1. Why can't we go now?
2. knows why	2. Who knows why?
3. guess why	3. I can guess why.
4. why don't	4. Why don't you tell us?
5. tell you why	5. I can't tell you why.

Phrases	*Sentences*
/traɪ/	
1. try to get	1. Try to get it right.
2. try again	2. I'll try again.
3. we'll try	3. We'll try to call her.
4. until you try	4. You won't know until you try.
5. try me	5. Try me first.
/draɪ/	
1. went dry	1. The well went dry.
2. dry your hands	2. Dry your hands well.
3. I'm dry	3. I'm dry—give me a drink.
4. hot and dry	4. It's sure hot and dry today.
5. drip dry	5. That's a drip dry shirt.
/kraɪ/	
1. don't cry	1. Don't cry about it.
2. could cry	2. I'm so mad I could cry.
3. a good cry	3. A good cry may help.
4. cry wolf	4. What does cry wolf mean?
5. cry baby	5. She's such a cry baby!
/flaɪ/	
1. to fly	1. I love to fly.
2. fly away	2. Let's fly away together.
3. shoo fly	3. Shoo, fly, don't bother me.
4. fly away	4. Fly away, little bird!
5. cheaper to fly	5. It's really cheaper to fly.
/skaɪ/	
1. sky is falling	1. Who said the sky is falling?
2. high as the sky	2. It's high as the sky.
3. sky diver	3. He's a sky diver.
4. blue as the sky	4. It's as blue as the sky.
5. sky is cloudy	5. The sky is cloudy today.

/aɪ/ CONTEXTS

Distinctive features: glide combination from /a/ to /ɪ/
/aɪ/ ***consonant combinations:*** Final position of an unstressed syllable

Deep Test

/maɪ/ myself

Common Words

/maɪ/

myself

Everyday Language

Phrases

/maɪ/

1. do it myself
2. all by myself
3. besides myself
4. myself today
5. shoot myself

Sentences

1. I'll do it myself.
2. I ate it all by myself.
3. There are two besides myself.
4. I was not myself today.
5. I think I'll shoot myself!

/aʊ/ CONTEXTS

Distinctive features: glide combination from /a/ to /ʊ/
/aʊ/ ***consonant combinations:*** Initial position of a stressed syllable

Deep Test

/aʊt/ out /aʊr/ our

Common Words

/aʊt/	/aʊr/
out	hour
outside	our
without	

Everyday Language

Phrases	*Sentences*
/aʊt/	
1. take it out	1. Take it out, please.
2. play outside	2. Let's play outside.
3. without you	3. We can't go without you.
4. you're out	4. Strike three, you're out!
5. without it	5. Try to do without it.
/aʊr/	
1. last an hour	1. It will last an hour.
2. an hour away	2. It's about an hour away.
3. our house	3. Our house is ready.
4. our place	4. Come over to our place.
5. our school	5. Our school won the game.

/aʊ/ CONTEXTS

Distinctive features: glide combination from /a/ to /ʊ/
/aʊ/ ***consonant combinations:*** Medial position of a stressed syllable

Deep Test

/maʊ/ amount	/raʊ/ around	/faʊ/ found	/klaʊ/ cloud
/daʊ/ doubt	/paʊ/ pound	/ʃaʊ/ shout	/kraʊ/ crowd
/kaʊ/ account	/baʊ/ about	/haʊ/ house	/graʊ/ ground
/saʊ/ sound	/taʊ/ town	/braʊ/ brown	

Common Words

/maʊ/	/daʊ/	/kaʊ/	/saʊ/	/raʊ/	/paʊ/	/baʊ/
amount	doubt	account	sound	around	pound	about
mount	down	count	south	round		
mountain						
mouth						

/taʊ/	/faʊ/	/ʃaʊ/	/haʊ/	/braʊ/	/klaʊ/	/kraʊ/
town	found	shout	house	brown	cloud	crowd

/graʊ/
ground

Everyday Language

Phrases	*Sentences*
/maʊ/	
1. small amount	1. That's a small amount.
2. mount up	2. Troubles mount up.
3. highest mountain	3. What is the highest mountain?
4. open your mouth	4. Just don't open your mouth!
5. close your mouth	5. Close your mouth, please.
/daʊ/	
1. doubt it	1. I doubt it.
2. feeling down	2. She's feeling down today.
3. down this way	3. It's down this way.
4. doubt him	4. Do you doubt him?
5. doubt about it	5. There's no doubt about it.
/kaʊ/	
1. my account	1. Put it on my account.
2. count on him	2. You can count on him.
3. this account	3. This account is overdue.
4. count them	4. Count them for me.
5. you count	5. Can you count to a million?
/saʊ/	
1. isn't a sound	1. There isn't a sound.
2. head south	2. Let's head south.
3. make a sound	3. Don't make a sound.
4. south of here	4. They live south of here.
5. down south	5. It's warm down south.
/raʊ/	
1. round and round	1. We went round and round.
2. around the corner	2. Around the corner is a place.
3. round them	3. Round them up now.
4. make it round	4. Make it round as you can.
5. around here	5. Do you live around here?
/paʊ/	
1. get a pound	1. Just get a pound.
2. lost a pound	2. I think I lost a pound!
3. pound it	3. Pound it down.
4. pound cake	4. Want some pound cake?
5. pound each	5. There's about a pound each.

Phrases	*Sentences*
/baʊ/	
1. all about	1. What's it all about?
2. about dogs	2. The story is about dogs.
3. about finished	3. I'm about finished.
4. about time	4. It's about time.
5. about four	5. About four, I'll go.
/taʊ/	
1. go to town	1. Let's go to town.
2. this town	2. This town is dead.
3. what town	3. What town is next?
4. small town	4. He's a small town boy.
5. home town	5. What's your home town?
/faʊ/	
1. found it	1. Who found it?
2. found her	2. He found her.
3. we found	3. We found it first.
4. lost is found	4. What's lost is found.
5. they found	5. They found nothing wrong.
/ʃaʊ/	
1. don't shout	1. Don't shout–I hear you!
2. have to shout	2. You'll have to shout.
3. shout out loud	3. Shout out loud to be heard.
4. someone shout	4. Did someone shout?
5. heard a shout	5. We heard a shout.
/haʊ/	
1. my house	1. My house is your house.
2. your house	2. Where is your house?
3. big house	3. It's the big house on the corner.
4. green house	4. Is it the green house?
5. white house	5. No, the white house next to it.
/braʊ/	
1. brown cow	1. How now brown cow.
2. brown is	2. Brown is a warm color.
3. brown coat	3. My brown coat is worn out.
4. brown dress	4. I'd like a brown dress.
5. brown bread	5. Brown bread is best.

Phrases	*Sentences*
/klaʊ/	
1. cloud in the sky	1. There isn't a cloud in the sky.
2. dark cloud	2. There's a dark cloud over there.
3. cloud up	3. It may cloud up today.
4. that cloud	4. That cloud is threatening.
5. rain cloud	5. It's a rain cloud.
/kraʊ/	
1. big crowd	1. There was a big crowd.
2. crowd me	2. Don't crowd me!
3. crowd up	3. We'll have to crowd up.
4. the crowd	4. The crowd has thinned out.
5. have a crowd	5. Hope we have a crowd!
/graʊ/	
1. lost ground	1. We lost ground on that.
2. the ground work	2. First lay the ground work.
3. ground level	3. It's at ground level.
4. ground or whole	4. Do you want it ground or whole?
5. ground beef	5. You'll need a pound of ground beef.

/aʊ/ CONTEXTS

Distinctive features: glide combination from /a/ to /ʊ/
/aʊ/ ***consonant combinations:*** Final position of a stressed syllable

Deep Test

/haʊ/ how /θaʊ/ thousand /naʊ/ now /laʊ/ allow /flaʊ/ flower
/paʊ/ power

Common Words

/haʊ/	/paʊ/	/θaʊ/	/naʊ/	/laʊ/	/flaʊ/
how	power	thousand	now	allow	flower

Everyday Language

Phrases	*Sentences*
/haʊ/	
1. how are	1. How are you today?
2. know how	2. I don't know how.
3. how can	3. How can you be sure?
4. how about	4. How about that!
5. not how	5. Not how, but when?
/paʊ/	
1. the power	1. Turn off the power.
2. takes power	2. That takes power.
3. power up	3. Let's power up now!
4. extra power	4. We'll need extra power.
5. more power	5. More power to you!
/θaʊ/	
1. a thousand	1. It's worth a thousand.
2. thousand times	2. A thousand times, No!
3. over a thousand	3. It's over a thousand now.
4. give a thousand	4. Who'd give a thousand?
5. thousand people	5. A thousand people came.
/naʊ/	
1. not now	1. Not now, please.
2. now is	2. Now is the time.
3. sorry now	3. Who's sorry now?
4. now you've	4. Now you've done it!
5. now and then	5. Now and then I do.
/laʊ/	
1. allow it	1. They won't allow it.
2. allow a little	2. Allow a little more time.
3. allow as how	3. I allow as how they would.
4. can allow	4. We can allow one more.
5. don't allow	5. Don't allow it to happen.
/flaʊ/	
1. as a flower	1. She's as pretty as a flower.
2. full flower	2. They're in full flower.
3. a flower	3. Send her a flower.
4. like a flower	4. It opens like a flower.
5. flower shop	5. He runs a flower shop.

/ɔɪ/ CONTEXTS

Distinctive features: glide combination from /ɔ/ to /ɪ/
/ɔɪ/ ***consonant combinations:*** Initial position of a stressed syllable

Deep Test

/ɔɪl/ oil

Common Words

/ɔɪl/
oil

Everyday Language

Phrases

/ɔɪl/

1. some oil
2. a little oil
3. vinegar and oil
4. oil changed
5. from oil

Sentences

1. You need some oil.
2. A little oil should help.
3. I'd like vinegar and oil.
4. Better have the oil changed.
5. Energy comes from oil.

/ɔɪ/ CONTEXTS

Distinctive features: glide combination from /ɔ/ to /ɪ/
/ɔɪ/ ***consonant combinations:*** Medial position of a stressed syllable

Deep Test

/pɔɪ/ point /dʒɔɪ/ join /vɔɪ/ voice /sɔɪ/ soil

Common Words

/pɔɪ/	/dʒɔɪ/	/vɔɪ/	/sɔɪ/
point	join	voice	soil

Everyday Language

Phrases	*Sentences*
/pɔɪ/	
1. the point	1. Well, what's the point?
2. sharp point	2. Make a sharp point.
3. point him out	3. Point him out to me.
4. don't point	4. Don't point; it's rude.
5. the point is	5. The point is, you can't.
/dʒɔɪ/	
1. join us	1. Come join us for dinner.
2. did you join	2. When did you join?
3. join the two	3. Join the two ends together.
4. join hands	4. All join hands and circle.
5. join anything	5. She'll join anything.
/vɔɪ/	
1. good voice	1. He has a good voice.
2. fine voice	2. You're in fine voice today.
3. just voice	3. Just voice your opinion.
4. the voice	4. It's the voice of the people.
5. my voice	5. I've lost my voice.
/sɔɪ/	
1. rich soil	1. That's rich soil.
2. soil your dress	2. Did you soil your dress?
3. top soil	3. It needs more top soil.
4. good soil	4. Good soil costs a lot.
5. potting soil	5. Do you have some potting soil?

/ɔɪ/ CONTEXTS

Distinctive features: glide combination from /ɔ/ to /ɪ/
/ɔɪ/ ***consonant combinations:*** Final position of a stressed syllable

Deep Test

/dʒɔɪ/ joy /bɔɪ/ boy /strɔɪ/ destroy

Common Words

/dʒɔɪ/	/bɔɪ/	/strɔɪ/
enjoy	boy	destroy
joy		

Everyday Language

Phrases	*Sentences*
/dʒɔɪ/	
1. enjoy it	1. I don't enjoy it.
2. great joy	2. There's great joy tonight!
3. enjoy yourself	3. Try to enjoy yourself.
4. joy to	4. Let's sing "Joy to the World."
5. she's a joy	5. She's a joy to have around.
/bɔɪ/	
1. good boy	1. He's a good boy.
2. boy or girl	2. Was it a boy or girl?
3. boy friend	3. Who's your boyfriend?
4. boy am	4. Boy, am I tired!
5. baby boy	5. They have a baby boy.
/strɔɪ/	
1. destroy him	1. The news will destroy him.
2. destroy it	2. A fire could destroy it.
3. destroy the world	3. They're going to destroy the world!
4. destroy the papers	4. Did they destroy the papers?
5. destroy the box	5. Don't destroy the box it came in.

INDEX

PHONEME		SYLLABLE POSITION					
Singles	Blends	Initial Stressed	Initial Unstressed	Medial Stressed	Medial Unstressed	Final Stressed	Final Unstressed
p	(p)	13 (18)	15			16 (19)	
b	(b)	20 (25)	23 (26)			24	
t	(t)	27 (35)	29			31 (36)	35
d		37	39			41	44
k	(k)	45 (53)	48			49 (54)	52 (55)
g	(g)	56 (61)	58			59	60
f	(f)	62 (67)	65			66 (68)	66
v		69	70			71	73
θ		74	75			76	
ð		77	79			80	
s	(s)	81 (90)	85 (92)			86 (93)	89 (94)
z		95	96			96	98
ʃ		99	101			102	104
ʒ		104					
h		105	108				
hw		109	110				
w		111	113				
l	(l)	114	117			119 (122)	121
r	(r)	125 (131)	127 (134)			129 (136)	(137)
j		138	140				
m		140	143			145 (148)	147 (149)

n		150	152			154 (158)	157 (160)
ŋ	ŋ					161 (164)	163
tʃ		164	166			167	
dʒ		169	170			171	172
i		173		174		180	
I		182	184	186	193		195
e		197		198		203	
ϵ		206		208			
æ		215	217	218			
ɑ		224		225	230		
ɔ		231	232	233		237	
o		238		240	245		248
U				249	251		
u				252	256	257	260
ɝ		260		261		263	
ɚ					265		266
ʌ		271		272			
ə			276		279		281
aI		285	286	287	291	292	296
aU		296		297		300	
ɔI		302		302		303	

TABLE III. Cross-references to *Sound Search II* software and *Sound Search: A Speech and Language Drillbook*

Sound Search II disks	*Sound groups*	*Sound Search drillbook* page reference
Module 1	/r/-/s/-/z/-/l/	125-81-95-114
Module 2	/p/-/b/-/t/-/d/-/k/-/g/	13-20-27-37-45-56
Module 3	/m/-/n/-/ŋ/-/f/-/v/-/θ/-/ð/	140-150-161-62-69-74-77
Module 4	/h/-/hw/-/w/-/j/	105-109-111-138
Module 5	/tʃ/-/dʒ/-/ʃ/-/ʒ/	164-169-99-104
Module 6	Vowels	173 through 276
Module 7	Diphthongs	285 through 302

Sound Search II software disks are available from Harding & Harris, Inc., P.O. Box 1599, Orem, Utah 84057 (801) 224-2014.

JERRY GRIFFITH received his Ph.D. in speech-language pathology from the University of Illinois in 1961. He has taught in university training programs for more than twenty years and serves as a consultant to public schools and clinical programs. He is a registered psychologist and presently is Director of Psychology Services, Sarah Bush Lincoln Health Center, a community hospital. The material in this publication is based on his study of the distributional features of speech and language and how they apply to the clinical management of communication disorders.

LYNN E. MINER received his Ph.D. in speech pathology from the University of Illinois in 1970. He has taught at Eastern Illinois University and Southern Methodist University and is currently Assistant Dean of the Graduate School and Director of Research Support at Marquette University. His research interests include computational linguistic approaches to communicative disorders. He has published and lectured extensively with his colleague, Jerry Griffith.